Slim Samurai

Unleash Your Weight-Loss Warrior Within

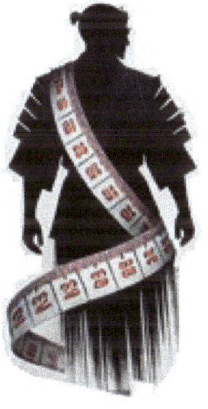

Tarek K.A. Hamid, PhD

Copyright ©2025 by Tarek K.A. Hamid

All rights reserved. No part of this book may be reproduced, stored in a retrieval system, or transmitted in any form or by any means—electronic, mechanical, photocopying, recording, or otherwise—without prior written permission from the author, except for brief quotations in reviews or as permitted by law.

Published by Metanoia Press Monterey, CA, 93953
Second Edition: March, 2025

Cover design by Jessica Bell Design

Printed in United States of America

ISBN: 979-8-9927562-0-3

Disclaimer: This book is intended for informational purposes only and should not be considered medical, nutritional, or professional advice. Readers should consult with a qualified healthcare provider before making any health or lifestyle changes.

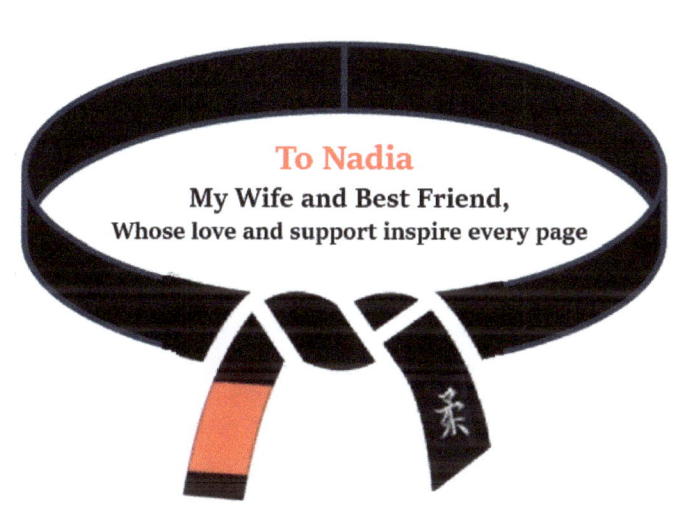

To Nadia
My Wife and Best Friend,
Whose love and support inspire every page

Contents

Prologue	1

Part I
The Struggle to Maintain a Healthy Weight:
And the Case for a Different Approach

Chapter 1 Looking Back … Before Moving Forward	21
2 The *Judo* Way	51
3 *Tsukuri:* We Can't Manage what we don't Understand	61

Part II
Judo-Inspired Weight-Loss Game Plan

Chapter 4 Managing Energy-In (Part A): *What* we Eat and Drink	99
5 Managing Energy-In (Part B): *How* we Eat and Drink	135
6 Exercising: Muscling the Body to Work *for us*	173
7 Beyond Physiology: The Challenges of Self-Regulation	193

Part III
Closing Argument: *Don't Delay*

Chapter 8 Time's Edge: Leverage it for Success	221
Index	233
Notes	235
About the Author	257

PROLOGUE

In 2021, the FDA's approval of *semaglutide* as an obesity medication, thrust the field of obesity treatment into a state of flux, upending longstanding conceptions and prompting reassessment of treatment strategies. (See sidebar.) This pivotal shift also inspired the writing of **Slim Samurai.**

> Ozempic and Wegovy are brand names for semaglutide, a medication originally approved by the FDA to treat type 2 diabetes. Both drugs, developed by the Danish pharmaceutical company Novo Nordisk, gained attention when clinical trials revealed semaglutide's effectiveness in reducing body weight. In June 2021, the FDA approved it for chronic weight management, marking a major milestone in the treatment of obesity and offering a new solution for those struggling with weight loss. Semaglutide works by mimicking GLP-1, a hormone that regulates appetite and food intake, and is administered via a weekly subcutaneous injection.
>
>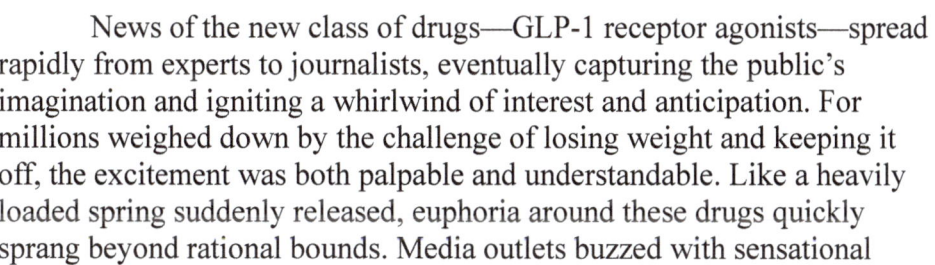

News of the new class of drugs—GLP-1 receptor agonists—spread rapidly from experts to journalists, eventually capturing the public's imagination and igniting a whirlwind of interest and anticipation. For millions weighed down by the challenge of losing weight and keeping it off, the excitement was both palpable and understandable. Like a heavily loaded spring suddenly released, euphoria around these drugs quickly sprang beyond rational bounds. Media outlets buzzed with sensational headlines and sweeping "mission accomplished" declarations.

It took some time for the frenzy to finally subside.

As the dust settled, a more discerning perspective emerged, fostering a sober and nuanced appreciation of the drugs' potential, limitations, and risks. David Ludwig, an obesity specialist and professor of pediatrics at Harvard Medical School, captured the broadening understanding of the drugs' strengths and shortcomings, remarking, "These drugs are potential game changers, but with an asterisk." They work by tamping down the body's hunger signaling pathways with an artificial sledgehammer—mimicking a hormone the intestine releases after eating that makes us feel full. However, they come with a long list of potential side effects, including serious digestive problems such as stomach paralysis, pancreatitis and bowel obstructions. Abruptly stopping the drugs can lead to rapid weight regain and worsen risk factors for diabetes and heart disease, according to a new standards of care report the American Diabetes Association's *Standards of Care in Diabetes—2025*. Furthermore, a significant portion of the weight lost with these drugs tends to come from lean muscle mass, which is far from ideal.[1]

A sampling of news headlines illustrates the media and public's journey from the dizzying heights of irrational exuberance to the grounded shores of rational discernment:

Euphoria: The Magic Bullet
- *AP (April, 2023): Powerful new obesity drug poised to upend weight loss care.*

- *PBS News Hour (Dec, 2023): Physician discusses surge in demand for weight-loss drugs.*

Reckoning: Costs and Risks
- *CNBC (April, 2024): Senate launches investigation into high prices of Ozempic and Wegovy.*

- *CNN (May, 2024): People using popular drugs for weight loss are more likely to be diagnosed with stomach paralysis… (and worse, see sidebar).*

Integration: One Tool in a Toolkit.
> *NPR (February, 2024): Weight-loss drugs aren't a magic bullet. Lifestyle changes are key to lasting health.*

> *NY Times (December, 2024): Blue Cross Blue Shield imposed new restrictions, including that some patients needed to prove they had participated in a lifestyle modification program to get coverage.*

And then there is… THE OZEMPIC FACE

Ozempic face is a popular phrase used to describe facial changes linked to rapid weight loss, particularly from using Ozempic. This pattern of rapid weight loss can lead to a reduction in facial fat, resulting in:

- A gaunt or hollowed-out appearance
- More prominent wrinkles or fine lines
- Sagging skin due to lost volume

However, ***Ozempic face*** is not a medical term. The use of this phrase risks trivializing a serious health condition and contributes to the growing list of negative memes associated with obesity.

Today, three years into the Ozempic era, a growing consensus among healthcare professionals affirms that lifelong health management still requires sustained commitment and meaningful lifestyle changes. While Ozempic can be a helpful companion on the weight-maintenance journey, it should not be relied on as the sole, singular strategy for weight management.[2] Instead, a holistic approach to personal health regulation—one that, as we'll discover, aligns closely with the core principles and foundational message of **Slim Samurai**—is essential.

It's important to recognize that this was, in fact, the FDA's intent all along. Back in 2021, the FDA's prescient approval statement read:

> *"Today (June 4, 2021), the U.S. Food and Drug Administration approved Wegovy (semaglutide) injection (2.4 mg once weekly) for*

*chronic weight management in adults with obesity or overweight with at least one weight-related condition (such as high blood pressure, type 2 diabetes, or high cholesterol), **for use in addition to a reduced calorie diet and increased physical activity***" (highlighting added).

Notably, even the manufacturers of these new drugs are now advocating for a more holistic approach. Likely spurred by recent research findings highlighting the risks of muscle loss and the development of frailty, especially in older patients, Novo Nordisk—the maker of Ozempic—launched an obesity prevention unit near Copenhagen in June 2023. This initiative aims to explore how lifestyle interventions can help "stop the disease before people turn to lifelong drugs to lose weight."

(Music to my ears! I'll be sure to send them a copy of **Slim Samurai**!)

The Upshot:

The development of the novel semaglutide-class weight-loss drugs represents a significant breakthrough, adding a powerful tool to our weight-loss toolkit and offering the potential for a reformation and reconceptualization of obesity treatment. However, a formidable challenge remains: persuading patients to use these drugs effectively and appropriately as part of a broader strategy, rather than viewing them as a standalone solution.

A major hurdle is overcoming our innate tendency to seek quick fixes and effortless solutions. The allure of the "silver bullet" is profoundly seductive, especially in a society where instant gratification reigns supreme. Weight-loss drugs like Ozempic are particularly appealing due to their simplicity—promising effortless weight loss with just a single injection once a week. Yet, is a lifelong weekly injection genuinely sustainable or desirable? That's the million-dollar question!

Many health professionals (this author included) believe the answer is probably no. Patients tend to dislike "forever" drugs, often due to a reluctance to take something that serves as a constant reminder of their illness. In the case of obesity drugs, factors such as side effects and cost issues can also contribute to discontinuation. A recent study at the Cleveland Clinic examined the electronic health records of 402 patients at sites in Ohio and Florida who were taking Wegovy or Ozempic for obesity. It found that only 161, or 40 percent, had consistently refilled their prescriptions over the course of the year. The researchers suggested that side effects, availability, or insurance and cost issues may have influenced these discontinuations.[3]

Reorienting individuals away from expedient pharmaceutical-only solutions, which may offer short-term relief but pose long-term risks, towards holistic and sustainable strategies is precisely the aim of **Slim Samurai**. Specifically, this book is intended for those who have used Ozempic and loved it but need to wean themselves off it, as well as for those who wish to avoid it or cannot afford it. It seeks to empower all of us—co-stakeholders in our increasingly obesogenic environment—to maintain lifelong healthy weights. *Sans* Ozempic.

As I will detail in the following chapters, the core thesis and prescriptive strategies of **Slim Samurai** align with the emerging holistic paradigm of personal health and weight regulation. They echo the conviction that it is not only the sustainable and healthy approach to long-term weight loss, but also key to obesity *prevention*. Which is paramount, since it is easier, less expensive, and more effective to change behavior so as to prevent weight gain, or to reverse small gains, than to treat obesity after it has fully developed.

In the remainder of this opening act, I will first outline the alarming scope of the obesity problem in modern society and underscore why *we are all at risk*. Next, I will present an overview of the book's novel approach, designed not only to help you shed those extra pounds but also to <u>maintain</u> a healthy weight over a lifetime.

A Sad Irony

For much of human history, body weight regulation was a piece of primeval cake. Humans didn't have to fuss about how much to eat to maintain a desirable body weight. Their bodies told them. For eons, feeding behavior was instinctively guided by biological signals indicating needs: eating when hungry (when the body signals an energy deficit) and stopping when full (when energy stores are replenished). Additionally, humans evolved taste buds that favored fat, salt, and sugar—nutrients that were relatively scarce yet essential for the body's proper functioning. In terms of both food quantity and quality, feeding behavior was essentially *ad-libitum*—literally meaning "at pleasure"—requiring little conscious effort.

Because obesity was not a prevalent health problem for most of human history, it is not surprising that humans have come to instinctively believe that their body's weight and energy regulation system is wisely *symmetric*—evenhandedly defending against both weight gain and loss while striving to maintain stability at a desirable body weight.[4] Unfortunately, this is a fundamental misconception and an increasingly risky one. In our modern obesifying environment, it lulls people into a false sense of invulnerability and seriously undermines obesity prevention efforts.

In reality, as I explain briefly below and in greater detail in Chapter 3, the body's energy regulation system is <u>not</u> evenhanded. Rather, it is *asymmetric*—favoring over-consumption rather than under-consumption and strongly defends against negative energy balance and weight loss. This design is no accident; it represents a beneficial evolutionary adaptation that equipped our hunter-gatherer ancestors with the drive to overeat (when food was plentiful) and efficiently store the excess energy as a buffer against future food shortages. And for eons, it worked—keeping them alive and in good shape in an environment where food was scarce and the next meal unpredictable.

It ain't working no more!

Today, we find ourselves in a paradoxical situation—simultaneously fortunate and unfortunate. In our modern, food-rich yet activity-poor environment, the very physiological adaptations that once helped our ancestors maintain good health are now leading to a maladaptive response: weight gain. Our pro-consumption physiology is still intact, still encouraging us to overeat. With constant access to high-calorie, high-fat foods and a sedentary lifestyle that limits opportunities for physical activity—whether at work, on the road, or at home—an imbalance between energy intake and output is increasingly prevalent across the population.[5] This scenario was not anticipated by biology, and given the human body's remarkable ability to adjust to excess calorie intake by storing body fat, the potential for weight gain today is significant.[6]

What a sad irony! The current environment of abundance and innovation that we toiled so hard to create, while a very comfortable one, is one that our body's energy-regulating system was not designed for. And an increasing number of people are paying a "heavy" price.[7]

It is essential to recognize that the technology-driven transformative leap of the last few centuries, constitutes but a mere evolutionary instant in the vast timeline of our species' evolutionary journey. A relatively swift pace of progress—in evolutionary terms—that outpaced our capacity to properly adapt. Not only physiologically, but I would argue behaviorally as well.

Evidence suggests that people remain bound not only by our Pleistocene-era physiology but also by démodé hunter-gatherer instincts that are ineffective in our present-day environment. For many, feeding behavior is largely instinctual and reflexive, driven more by cues of hunger and satiety, as well as external stimuli, than by conscious thought. This drives many of us—as it did to our hunter-gatherer ancestors—to eat to our physiological limits when food is abundant and to gravitate toward energy-dense foods.

The inevitable result?

In the span of just a few generations, the prevalence of overweightness among American adults has risen to an alarming 75%—this, according to the latest assessment by the Centers for Disease Control and Prevention (CDC). Even more concerning, close to half of those deemed overweight (that's approximately 100 million Americans) are now heavy enough to count as clinically obese—with a body mass index (BMI) greater than 30. (A BMI of 30—calculated as weight in kilograms divided by the square of the height in meters—roughly means being 30 pounds overweight for an average-height woman and 35 to 40 pounds overweight for an average-weight man.) That's being so overweight that their lives will likely be cut seriously shorter by excess fat.

The problem is no longer confined to America. The situation is nearly as dismal around the globe, as country after country follows the American lead and grows heavier.[8] Indeed, the World Obesity Federation is now predicting that by 2030, one billion people—one in five women and one in seven men—will be living with obesity.

It seems hard to believe that a health condition like obesity could spread with the speed and breadth of a communicable disease epidemic.[9] But it has.

Clearly, overweightness is not increasing because people are consciously trying to gain weight. One of the major perplexities of this condition is that more and more people are gaining weight even in the face of broad publicity about the problem, tremendous pressure to be thin and a titanic struggle by tens of millions of people to manage their weight. The billions of dollars Americans spend each year on weight-loss products and services further indicate that many are dissatisfied with the current state of affairs.

So, how then did we get into this predicament? And how could such an easily discernible problem sneak up on us so?

Maladaptation to Slow-building Threats… *in frogs and men*!

As the population's weight and waistlines steadily increased in the latter half of the last century, most public health experts and the general public failed to recognize the growing threat. In hindsight, it's easy to understand why. Unlike traditional infectious diseases such as malaria, tuberculosis, or COVID-19, obesity presents no immediate harmful symptoms. At first, it affected only a small portion of the population, and the rise in overweight and obese individuals was gradual enough that society had time to normalize it.[10]

On a personal level, weight gain also seems insidious to most people. Unlike the polar bear, people don't get fat by voracious fat eating in a short period. Instead, weight gain typically occurs slowly, over decades. For example, the age-related upward drift in weight for adult men is, on average, only about half a pound per year.[11] Because of a lack of immediate adverse consequences, the early stages of weight gain often go unnoticed or may be viewed as innocuous and inevitable, or even as a sign of maturity.[12] And so, a gradual increase in body weight might not be recognized until people are trapped in an unhealthy lifestyle, which can ultimately result in chronic obesity.

Maladaptation to slowly building threats—both at the personal and societal levels—is by no means limited to weight gain, and neither is it uncommon.

Human beings are exquisitely adapted to recognize and respond to threats to survival that come in the form of sudden, salient events. We're here today, as a species, because when something went bump in the night in the primeval forest, we noticed and reacted.[13] This fixation on sharp, jarring events is often seen as part of our evolutionary wiring.[14] Change that is slow and gradual, however, is less perceptible to our cognitive apparatus. This is why we're less likely to notice the signs of aging in someone we see every day, like a spouse or parent, but more likely to spot them in people we encounter only occasionally, such as distant relatives. It's not that we're incapable of detecting slow, continuous change; we often do, like when a perceptive fisherman reads shifts in cloud patterns signaling an approaching storm. But because our attention is finite—and life's events constantly compete for it—we tend to focus only on changes we deem urgent or threatening.[15] In the case of weight-gain, a lack of immediate adverse consequences often means that it is off our RADAR screen.

Maladaptation to creeping threats has been so pervasive and enduring in human affairs that it has been enshrined in social and public policy circles as the parable of the *boiled frog*.

> If you place a frog in a pot of boiling water, it will immediately try to scramble out. But if you place the frog in room temperature water, and don't scare him, he'll stay put. Now, if the pot sits on a heat source, and if you gradually turn up the temperature, something very interesting happens. As the temperature rises from 70 to 80 degrees Fahrenheit, the frog will do nothing. In fact, he will show every sign of enjoying himself. As the temperature gradually increases, the frog will become groggier and groggier, until he is unable to climb out of the pot. Though

there is nothing restraining him, the frog will sit there and boil. Why? Because the frog's internal apparatus for sensing threats to survival is geared to sudden changes in his environment, not to slow, gradual changes.[16]

The parable aims to illustrate how subtle, gradual changes—no matter how harmful—can go unnoticed and tolerated over time, ultimately leading to disaster for the unaware or complacent.

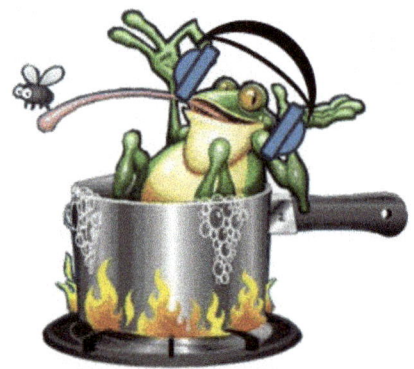

But, hold on—you'd be rightful to demur—while frogs (and perhaps hunter-gatherers) may guilelessly succumb to a slow boil, surely, *we* wouldn't. Certainly, not in today's information age?

It stands to reason that in this era of technology and instant information, today's tech-savvy *Homo Digitalis* would know better than to stay in the metaphorical boiling pot. But think again! One of the great ironies of America's obesity epidemic is that at a time when Americans arguably know more about food and nutrition than at any time in their history, we are gaining more weight. (As I've attempted to intimate by the earphone-adorning <u>boiling</u> frog in the above cartoon!) Despite all the diet books, the wide availability of low-calorie and low-fat foods, and the broad publicity about the obesity problem, the epidemic continues to grow at a rate that rivals or exceeds that of forty years ago.[17, 18]

The persistence and pervasiveness of the problem may surprise many and frustrate policy makers, but it is no mystery to cognitive psychologists.

The Power—and traps—of Emotions and Self-serving Delusions

> *Many of us use information as a drunken man uses lampposts –*
> *for support rather than for illumination.*
>
> Andrew Wang[19]

A wealth of research in behavioral decision-making has demonstrated that our thinking is influenced not solely by logic and information processing, but also by the influence of ingrained beliefs and/or self-serving interpretations. For instance, people often unconsciously seek out information that confirms their preexisting views, while avoiding information that challenges them—a tendency known as confirmation bias.[20] It's why access to more information tends to increase *confidence* in judgment—people assume that the quality of decisions has improved because they can find information to support them—but it does not necessarily increase the *quality* of judgment.[21]

Needs and emotions also weigh heavily into the social judgment process, and people's expectations often correspond closely with what they would *like* to see happen or to what is socially desirable rather than to what is objectively likely.[22] A clear example is the widespread unrealistic optimism about health risks. People consistently demonstrate what psychologists call the "illusion of unique invulnerability," believing they are less likely than others to experience injury or negative health outcomes. This "it won't happen to me" mindset has been observed across a broad spectrum of diseases, hazards, and disasters. Research in clinical and developmental psychology suggests that such positive illusions fulfill various cognitive, emotional, and social functions. For example, unrealistic optimism about health risks is often an attempt to avoid the anxiety one would feel from admitting a threat to well-being—a form of defensive denial. Illusions about unique invulnerability can also enhance a person's self-esteem. In problems like overweightness or drug addiction, which many believe to be caused by behavior or personality, people may feel invulnerable because they would like to believe that they do not have the weakness of character that allows it to develop *in them*.[23]

While the capacity to develop and maintain positive illusions—about oneself or one's loved-ones—may help make each individual's world a warmer place in which to live, it can be a risky business. Unrealistic optimism in matters of health and disease often leads people to ignore legitimate risks in their environment and avoid taking the necessary measures to offset those risks.[24] This, of course, can become a significant impediment to preventing conditions such as weight gain. If people convince themselves that they are invulnerable to weight gain, then they are unlikely to take measures to reduce their risk of gaining weight no matter how educated they are about the dire consequences of excessive body weight. The it won't happen to me mindset gets in their way: why protect yourself from an event that will not occur?

For individuals who are already overweight, another self-serving distortion that evades reality is body-weight *mis-*assessment. Numerous studies have shown significant discrepancies between individuals' perceptions of their weight and their actual weight status. In one of the most referenced studies, researchers sought to assess the degree of agreement between individuals' *actual* weight status, as measured by their body mass index (BMI), and their *perceptions* of their weight status. Sifting through data from the third National Health and Nutrition Examination Survey (NHANES III, 1988-94)—one of several large-scale national surveys conducted by the Centers for Disease Control and Prevention (CDC) between 1960 and 2004—they found that large segments of the U.S. population had a distorted perception of their weight status, and not just by small margins—such as weights being just a few pounds over the overweight threshold—but often by substantial amounts. (Notably, overweight men were the primary offenders, with 43 percent of overweight male participants mistakenly believing they were of average weight or underweight.[25])

Even more concerning is the finding that parents of overweight children often underestimate their children's weight.[26] For instance, one study revealed that only 21% of mothers with overweight preschool children recognized their child as overweight.[27]

These misperceptions about weight have clear implications for how individuals perceive risk—both for themselves and their children.

Which, most health experts agree, pose significant obstacles to prevention efforts.

Socio-Climate Change… and the Risk we all Face

> *"Humans have constructed the most sophisticated civilization ever to grace the planet, but countless millions need to medicate themselves to cope with living within them."*
> Brian Klaas[28]

The torrent of obesogenic pressures in our modern environment has often been likened to fast and furious sea currents sweeping *all* ships out to sea. It is an apt metaphor. These pressures disrupt our energy balance by increasing calorie intake and reducing energy expenditure, steadily raising body weights across society. (Interestingly, as with the environmental drivers of obesity—which I am characterizing as *socio*-climate change—scientists note that the intensity of tidal currents has also risen in recent years due to climate change.)

Our physical and social environments provide us with the context in which to live our lives—what we eat and how we work, play, and move around, all of which affect energy intake and expenditure. What we decide to eat is not only a matter of personal preferences, but also very much a function of what food is available in the variety of food outlets we have access to in our communities. Similarly, our choices concerning physical activity are simultaneously a function of lifestyle choices and the characteristics of our environment.

Here is a sampling of *socio*-climate pressures—on both sides of the human energy balance equation—that most of us would be familiar with from daily life experiences:

- Obesogenic pressures increasing *energy-intake*:
    - Overabundance of convenient energy-dense fatty foods
    - Diminishing affordability of healthful foods

- o Growing trend towards larger portion sizes—in restaurants and at home (e.g., of packaged foods and soft drinks).

- Obesogenic pressures decreasing *energy-expenditure*:
  - o Modern labor-saving technologies in the farm, factory, office.
  - o Widespread diffusion of screen-based leisure activities—such as television, video games, and internet browsing—that foster sedentary lifestyles.
  - o Automobile-centric urban designs of cities, towns, and suburbs that discourage non-motorized transportation, such as walking and biking.

Living in a world of high-calorie, high-fat foods, always in plentiful supply, and with labor-saving devices that keep us from having to exert ourselves too much, our wired-in energy-regulatory processes sometimes fail us. They tell us to eat more than we need for a healthy, normal weight, and, if we listen to their signals, we get fat.

Analogous to mighty sea currents that sweep unsuspecting swimmers (and ships) out to sea, the mismatch between our body's asymmetric system of weight-energy regulation and our modern obesifying environment means *we are all at risk*.

This makes maintaining a healthy weight in our modern environment a very different matter than it was intended to be. Rather than being an unconscious and automatic process, it has become something we must actively manage. Our dilemma lies in finding ways to sustain a healthy weight without advocating for a regression in societal progress. For example, it would be undesirable, as well as infeasible, to attempt to engineer physical activity back into our modern, non-labor-intensive jobs—whether on factory floors or in the fields.[29]

Thankfully, such drastic measures may not be necessary. Maintaining a healthy weight is certainly achievable without sacrificing the modern conveniences we've worked so hard to attain. However, as I argue in *Slim Samurai*, devising effective, sustainable strategies for lifelong weight management—not just for a week or a month, but for a lifetime—requires a fundamental shift in thinking. This novel approach involves working with our body's wired-in physiological processes rather than fight against them. The aim of this book is to show you how.

Book's Plan

The immense effort and expense that millions invest in weight management suggest that the struggle to lose weight—and keep it off—is not due to a lack of *will* but rather a lack of *skill*. Specifically, it reflects inadequate understanding of the machinations of the body's energy regulation system and, consequently, a failure to devise *sustainable* strategies that effectively counteract its inherent asymmetric defenses.

In *Slim Samurai*, we will begin by building your weight and energy regulation *skill*. Specifically, the aim is to enhance your conceptual understanding of the weight-energy regulation system so you are better able to formulate effective weight-loss strategies that align with your personal health needs and lifestyle preferences. More concretely, help you devise high-leverage strategies that work with your body's wired-in physiological processes rather than against them. It's a novel—*Judo*-inspired—approach to personal health regulation.

Next, we'll explore a repertoire of proven, *maximum-efficiency, minimum-effort* strategies than can help you better regulate energy intake and expenditure. These tactics are adaptable, allowing you to adjust the intensity—dialing it up or down—as needed to lose weight in the short term or to maintain a healthy weight over the long term in a food-rich activity-poor environment. Much like a swimmer who may need only gentle strokes to hold position in a steady current but must exert more effort to backpedal if swept into deeper waters, the weight-regulation techniques we'll examine are essentially the same whether you're aiming to lose or sustain weight. While the level of intensity may change, the "strokes" remain fundamentally the same.

Perhaps most importantly, these max-efficiency, min-effort strategies are designed to be simple to integrate into daily life and comfortable enough to sustain over the long term. In today's environment, where unhealthy habits are easy to adopt and hard to avoid, maintaining a healthy weight will demand consistent effort and lifelong vigilance. Just as a swimmer wouldn't—or shouldn't—float idly in a strong current, we can't rely on "automatic cruise control" for our eating and activity habits in today's obesogenic world. Long-term weight maintenance is a lifelong project, and these adaptable, Judo-inspired tactics can help you navigate it effectively.

The book is divided into three parts. *Part I* lays the conceptual foundation for the rest of the text. In Chapter 1, I provide a deeper discussion of the challenging obesity problem, its burden, and the need for a *different* approach. Chapter 2 presents the argument for the Judo-inspired strategy. Before moving on to a discussion of the nuts-and-bolts of the Judo-esque weight-loss game-plan, Chapter 3 is a preparatory "go to school" chapter on the workings of the human weight and energy regulation system. The goal is to gain a better understanding of how this complex system operates—specifically, how processes like energy consumption and expenditure are interconnected and influenced by the external environment. Understanding how and why the system behaves the way it does and what effects our interventions will or will not have is essential in identifying *leverage* points in the system and, thus, in devising appropriate strategies for change.

The focus of *Part II* is on the game-plan. Chapters 4 and 5 focus on tactics relating to *what* and *how* we eat, i.e., on *energy-in*. The second limb of the energy equation is *energy out*—physical activity and exercising—and is the focus of Chapter 6. In Chapter 7 we extend the Judo principles of "maximum efficiency – minimum effort" to the *cognitive* domain, specifically how to set weight-loss goals and effectively regulate your self-control energy to stay the course. We'll learn that, just as in the realm of physical energy, the *seiryoku zenyo* principle of maximum efficiency is equally applicable to the exercise of mental energy. And just as effective. Specifically, we will understand that our self-regulatory capacity, which is crucial for successful long-term weight-loss maintenance, is an invaluable yet limited resource that needs to be *efficiently* managed and must not be squandered.

Having discussed the tactics for managing weight gain and loss, I conclude in *Part III* (Chapter 8) by emphasizing that *when* we act is just as important. I argue that economy of means is not just about *how* we accomplish things, but is also very much a function of *when* we act.

Indeed, the how and the when are inextricably linked, since what we can or cannot do now is often constrained by decisions we've already made. When it comes to health regulation and weight gain, it is crucial to intervene before the cumulative burden of bad behavior escalates to the point where it becomes exceedingly difficult to reverse the damage. Acting without delay, in essence, *makes it less hard for the body to work for us.*

Part I

The Struggle to Maintain Healthy Weight: And the Case for a Different Approach

The fact that millions of people struggle to lose weight and keep it off, despite investing significant time, money, and effort, suggests that lasting weight loss is not a matter of *will* but of *skill*.

A primary goal of *Slim Samurai* is to help you develop the *skills* needed for effective weight and energy regulation. Specifically, the aim is to deepen your conceptual understanding—your mental model, if you will—of the complex human weight-energy regulation system enabling you to skillfully design effective weight-loss strategies that align with your unique health needs and lifestyle preferences. More concretely, *Slim Samurai* guides you in crafting *Judo-inspired* high-leverage strategies that work with, rather than against, your body's wired-in physiological processes. Not only to lose weight but to sustain it for the long term.

Before delving into the day-to-day weight-loss strategies of Part II, Part I lays essential groundwork for meaningful change. This section focuses on building the intellectual and emotional foundation needed for a true mindset shift, exploring how we think about our bodies, weight regulation, and the nature of personal transformation. It's a discussion that ventures into more philosophical—and perhaps even unsettling—territory as it challenges widely held misconceptions. Yet, this exploration is vital, encouraging you to jettison outdated beliefs about health and self-regulation and paving the way for lasting success in your journey.

Chapter 1 serves as a diagnostic, looking back—and around—to uncover deeply entrenched misconceptions about weight and energy regulation that may be hindering your weight-management efforts. The notion of looking back before moving forward is rooted in many Eastern philosophical traditions, including Confucianism, Daoism, and Buddhism, which emphasize mindfulness and reflection on past choices (and missteps) to inform future actions and foster growth and enlightenment.

After this diagnostic reflection, Chapter 1 closes by advocating for a shift in approach. As Albert Einstein observed, "The significant problems we face cannot be solved at the same level of thinking we were at when we created them"—we need to adopt a deeper level of thinking to address these challenges.

Chapter 2 argues for and introduces the novel Judo-inspired approach to weight and energy regulation and outlines the philosophical principles that underpin the *Judo way*. At its core, Judo's philosophy emphasizes understanding one's opponent—identifying their strengths and weaknesses—before engaging. In this spirit, Chapter 3 will guide us in studying the intricacies of the human weight and energy regulation system before we dive into the Judo-inspired strategies of Part II. This understanding is essential for developing effective, high-leverage strategies that work with the body's natural processes.

Chapter 1

Looking Back ... Before Moving Forward

If you're still reading (😊), it's likely because you're either hesitant to try Ozempic or have tried it, found it effective, but now feel ready—or even compelled—to move beyond it. By picking up this book, you're signaling an interest—perhaps even an eagerness—to explore alternative, sustainable strategies for achieving lifelong healthy weight, free from reliance on Ozempic.

If that sounds like you, let's dive in.

Many of us approach weight regulation as we would a boxing match—seeking a swift and decisive knockout of a tough and obstinate foe: our own body. The record to-date has been pretty clear: few of us can land that decisive knockout punch. (As we'll explore, the reasons lie more in our physiology than in psychology or willpower.) In *Slim Samurai*, I argue that we'd have a much better shot if we approach the weight-regulation fight differently—using the deft and more efficient strategies of the *Judo wrestler*. Not only to lose weight but also to prevent regaining it.

Judo, arguably the most scientific of the martial arts, teaches the value and tactics of gaining advantage over a formidable opponent by using leverage, balance, and, most ingeniously, the transfer of power—redirecting an opponent's own force and momentum against them, rather than opposing it directly. If the opponent pushes you pull, if pulled you push. It has long been touted as the most effective (and even wily) strategy to defend oneself against larger and stronger opponents.

In the following chapters, I aim to demonstrate both the utility and feasibility of deploying judo-esque tactics that *work with our body* not against it, to successfully lose weight and keep it off. But before I ask you to swap your metaphorical—and possibly worn-out—boxing gloves for a *Judogi* uniform, it behooves us to first take a look back to try and understand why current weight-regulation schemes have not been… well knockouts? And probably never will. And contemplate the costs—and risks—of staying the course. As the saying goes, how much we learn from our failures determines how far we go in achieving our goals.[30]

It's Difficult to Resist a *K.I.S.S.*

Cognitive theorists and philosophers have long argued that humans instinctively seek simple explanations—and, by extension, simplistic solutions—for even the most complex problems. This explains why so-called *KISS*—Keep It Simple, Stupid—solutions are widely appealing, even seductive. Confronting a knotty problem or situation can be both emotionally and cognitively taxing, which is why it is understandable that people often gravitate toward simplistic characterizations and uncomplicated remedies. But as Harvard economist John Kenneth Galbraith—who coined the phrase "conventional wisdom"—warned, while simplistic views may be convenient and comforting, they aren't necessarily accurate.[31] He argued that people often cling to these simplifications, like a raft in rough waters, simply because they're easier to manage than the full, intricate reality.

Personal health and body weight regulation is a good case in point.

Instructions for losing weight in self-help books cannot be simpler. They go something like this: induce a weekly caloric deficit of 3,500 calories—through either dieting or exercise—and you'll lose one pound in a week, ten pounds in ten weeks. The underlying assumptions being that the there is a fixed energy cost of 3,500 calories per pound of lost tissue, and that the relationship is linear—meaning that if the diet is maintained, weight drops in an uninterrupted straight-line fashion.

Both these assumptions, as we'll see, are *wrong*.

For instance, the energy cost of lost tissue is *not* fixed at 3,500 kcal/lb. since tissue loss is never 100 percent pure fat. Rather, it is always a combination of both fat mass (FM) and fat-free mass (FFM)—the relative composition depending, in part, on the person's initial body composition. Because fat and lean tissue are *not* energetically equivalent, the energy content of a pound of lost tissue varies among people and even for the same person over time.

Furthermore, that simplistic assumption of linearity leads to absurd weight loss projections—suggesting, for example, that one could lose 50 pounds in a year or nearly 150 pounds over three years!

In reality, losing weight is not that straightforward. Weight loss typically slows over time—even if the prescribed diet *is* strictly followed—and people tend to lose less weight than prescribed... much less. It's primarily because when weight is lost as a result of caloric restriction, involuntary homeostatic processes hardwired into our physiology kick in to conserve energy and lower energy expenditure in order to protect the body's energy reserves and restrain the rate of tissue depletion. (We'll delve deeper into the *why* and the *how* later.)

Figure 1.1 contrasts the naive conception of weight-loss dynamics with the frustrating reality that many exasperated dieters have experienced. Which goes something like this: after a brief initial phase of gratifying losses, the rate of weight loss invariably tapers off and ultimately body weight stabilizes at a level significantly higher than hoped for. Weight loss during prolonged caloric restriction is, thus, not the straightforward linear decline that most people expect, and count on; instead, it follows a *curvilinear* pattern, as illustrated in the figure.[32,33,34]

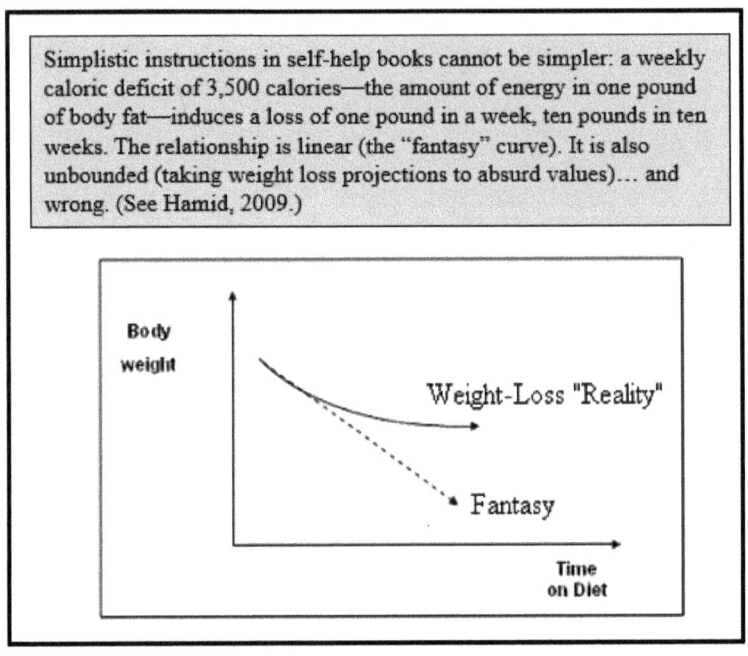

Figure 1.1
Weight-loss fantasy versus reality

Overlooking the body's energy-sparing mechanisms, which work to limit tissue loss during caloric deprivation, may sell more diet books, but it inevitably leads to spurious predictions of treatment outcomes. Which should be of concern, because people's expectations about treatment outcomes and the degree to which they are met or not met can significantly influence their self-efficacy, or belief in their ability to achieve their goals, and in turn long-term motivation and commitment.[35]

The prevalence and scale of the fantasy-reality gap among dieters has been striking—and consistently so—in experimental studies. In one notable example, a group of overweight women enrolled in a weight-loss program was asked to set their desired target weights before starting. On average, their target weights represented an ambitious 32 percent reduction from their starting weight. The reality? Nearly a year later, the average weight loss was only halfway to their goals, with almost half of the women failing to achieve even the weight loss level they had stated would be considered disappointing before starting treatment.[36]

While the failure to achieve desired levels of weight loss is a common frustration for dieters, what many find even more discouraging is the difficulty of maintaining even modest weight losses. The record shows that the majority of dieters who successfully lose (some) weight eventually regain it, typically reclaiming one to two-thirds of the lost weight within a year and nearly all of it—if not more—within five years.[37,38,39] Given the immense cultural pressure to be thin, however, this seldom dissuades people from trying again and again, often trapping them in a vicious cycle of weight loss and regain.

Which begs the question: why? Why do peddled be-all-and-end-all diets, which seem to pop up like a dime a dozen, never seem to be... well, knockouts? And, more importantly, why do we keep falling for them? Not once or twice, but time and time again.

I argue that this is due to two fundamental misconceptions. The first has to do with the aforementioned self-serving *under*-estimation of the complexity of the problem at hand and the second is an *over*-estimation of our capacity to learn from failure.

Simplistic Conceptions and KO Solutions that Rarely Score

Weight-gain is one of the most complex—and therefore misunderstood—human conditions, and perhaps as a result, it is one of the most exploited.[40,41] The obese and the overweight—which is now most of us—are pummeled with bad advice and patronized with marketing campaigns. Only the marketing has paid off! The weight-loss industry—which in 2015 generated more than $150 billion in the US and Europe—thrives for two reasons: selling promising knock-out (KO) remedies and repeat customers. The bold promises draw the customers in the first place, while the be-all-end-all illusory solutions virtually guarantee that they cannot be fulfilled. It makes for a very attractive business model!

KO-type solutions are an easy-sell not only because they are viscerally appealing, but also because they seem entirely plausible. Traditionally, when we recognize a problem, we reflect on it, devise a plan to address it, and then act on the plan, believing we have resolved the issue. For example: I can't sleep → I take a sleeping pill → Zzzz! For myriad routine everyday tasks, this intuitive *problem* → *action* → *end-of-story* scheme is indeed all it takes to get the job done (Figure 1.2).

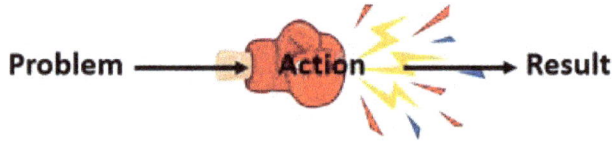

Figure 1.2 Knock-out

Until it doesn't!

When tackling complex, persistent problems, this circumscribed straight-line model is often a gross simplification of how reality works. Persistent problems—body weight and energy regulation being a perfect example—are challenging for a reason: *they fight back*! By that I mean, our interventions to change or correct the state of a system (such as our body weight), often trigger compensating feedback effects (called *homeostatic* processes in the case of human physiology) that resist—or even reverse—those changes. This explains why, even when it feels like we've successfully resolved (and are done with) a complex problem, *the problem is rarely done with us!*

This vexatious characteristic of complex systems to fight back is by no means limited to biology or human weight-energy regulation. Indeed, it characterizes many complex systems, whether physical, biological or social. (See sidebar for non-health-related example familiar to many of us: "traffic congestion.")

> ### System Fight-Back... and the experience of long-term pain after short-term gain
>
> System resistance to policy intervention is an often-encountered phenomenon in the public policy domain, where well-intentioned interventions offer immediate relief that prove ephemeral. A classic example is the building of roads to relieve congestion. When new roads are built, congestion level does indeed drop short run because it takes time for people's driving habits to adjust to the improved driving conditions. Inevitably, however, people adjust to the shorter travel times by driving more. It's called: *induced demand*—economist-speak for the observed phenomena where an increase in the supply of something (like roads) makes people want even more of it... albeit after some delay. The all-too-familiar result: few years after new roads are built or a highway is widened, the reduction in congestion leads to more trips and more cars, swiftly building congestion back up.

The (annoying) boomerang effect often comes as a shocking surprise. But that's almost always because our understanding of the problem is often incomplete or inaccurate. In the case of weight regain, for instance, this surprise often stems from the fact that most dieters don't fully grasp the complex array of homeostatic processes that regulate the human weight and energy system.

The human body relies on various homeostatic mechanisms to maintain internal stability, regulating processes such as body temperature, blood pressure, blood sugar, iron concentration, and energy reserves. (Homeostatic processes are self-regulating mechanisms by which systems—biological, mechanical, or social—work to maintain stability in response to environmental changes or external disruptions.) In the case of dieting, efforts to alter the body's state—specifically, to reduce tissue and deplete fat reserves—trigger compensatory energy conservation measures that aim to protect the body's energy stores. (A brief explanation of the *why* is provided in the next section, with a more detailed discussion of the *how* in Chapter 3.)

To be fair to dieters—as well as policymakers and city planners—such *homeostatic-type* counteractions can be difficult to anticipate and forestall. One important reason for this is the significant asymmetry in the delays between actions and reactions. It often takes much less time for an action to produce its intended result than it does for the system to mobilize a response. As a result, while the immediate effects of our actions are usually clear and directly observable, the secondary homeostatic effects are typically delayed by months— or, in cases like traffic congestion, even years. This delay makes it challenging to mentally close the loop (e.g., from congestion to more highway lanes, and back to re-congestion—the metaphorical "counterpunch"). In the case of human energy and weight regulation, opaqueness creates an additional complication. The metabolic-related homeostatic mechanisms that resist our weight-loss interventions are physiologic processes occurring inside our bodies, making them doubly hard to discern.

The antidote to boomerang effects or "counterblow" surprises? In the case of the human weight and energy regulation, it lies in developing a more complete and accurate understanding of the system—homeostatic processes, delays and all. In the next section, we dig a bit deeper into the physiological reasons why the body *fights* back against weight-loss efforts. And why, even after successfully losing weight, the challenge is far from over. Not by a long shot!

Like most Fights, it is Precipitated by a Misunderstanding

While the body's fightback to preserve its fat reserves might seem diabolical to exasperated dieters, in truth, it is neither mysterious nor capricious. Let's not forget, we are the only species on the planet in which hungry individuals will voluntarily refuse to consume readily available, appealing food in order to meet some aesthetic or health goals.[42,43] This is a distinctly modern phenomenon, one that nature never anticipated. Throughout human history, food deprivation has ordinarily been the result of ecological scarcity. Hence, our built-in physiologic defenses in response to food deprivation are the body's attempt to survive in the face of food scarcity. There was simply no evolutionary reason for our bodies to anticipate (or be designed for) *self-imposed* deprivation.

So, ...

In dieting, when any significant weight is lost, the loss is interpreted by the body as a deprivation crisis that needs to be contained... and is. To restrain the rate of tissue depletion, the body compensates by slowing its metabolism. This is achieved chiefly through hormonal mechanisms that operate to decrease the metabolic activity at the cellular level. This adjustment essentially enhances the body's metabolic efficiency—much like switching a home's light bulbs to fluorescent ones to save energy.[44] (Muscle biopsies taken before, during and after weight loss show that once a person drops weight, their muscle fibers undergo a transformation, making them more like highly efficient slow twitch muscle fibers that burn 20 to 25 percent fewer calories during everyday activity.[45]) Additionally, as weight is lost and both fat and fat-free tissue are shed, the body's maintenance energy requirements—the energy needed to support essential physiological functions and sustain cells—also decrease, simply because there's now less tissue to maintain. The combined effect of these two energy conservation measures is to effectively shrink the dieter's diet-induced energy deficit, which in turn (and unfortunately for the dieter) curbs the rate of weight loss and causes people to lose less weight than they expect... much less.

As an example, consider a hypothetical 160-pound overweight female whose steady-state caloric intake to maintain her weight is 2,000 kcal/day. Determined to lose weight, she decides to cut her daily intake to 1,500 kcal, creating an initial caloric deficit of 500 calories per day (2,000 - 1,500), or 3,500 calories per week. Her (naïve) expectation: to lose twelve pounds in three months. Unbeknownst to her, after several weeks on this diet and some initial weight loss, her body's energy needs adjust, decreasing from the pre-diet level of 2,000 calories to, say, 1,800 calories. Consequently, her daily energy deficit—the gap between her intake and the now-lowered energy expenditure—shrinks from 500 to 300 calories (1,800 - 1,500), a significant 40 percent reduction. Her body's involuntary energy conservation mechanisms thus effectively shrink her diet-induced energy deficit, slowing her rate of weight loss and leaving her short of her original goal.

The body's *involuntary* energy-sparing adaptations have both short- and long-term consequences. Short-term, they restrain the rate of tissue loss and mean that people tend to lose less weight than they expect. But because the body's fightback persists after caloric deprivation ends, there is the additional long-term risk of weight regain.

A recent Australian study sheds light on this long-term dynamic. In the groundbreaking research, a group of 50 overweight men and women completed a weight-loss program and were then monitored for many additional months to assess the long-term effects post-intervention. The findings were striking: participants remained in what could be described as a biologically altered state *for an entire year* after achieving significant weight loss. These persisting biological changes revealed why participants, like many dieters, continued to experience heightened hunger and depressed energy expenditure well after the intervention ended. Their still-plump bodies were acting as if they were still in a state of deprivation, working overtime to regain the pounds they lost.[46]

The body's *persistent intransigence* long after weight-loss interventions would matter less if our capacity for self-control were inexhaustible. But it is not. As discussed in detail in Chapter 7, experimental studies show that our ability for self-regulation—our capacity to resist temptations, persevere to finish tiring tasks, and so on—functions much like a muscle. And, just like muscular strength, it is not an inexhaustible resource. Thus, while determined dieters might be able to shed large amounts of weight by severely restricting their intake or even starving themselves for weeks, they will invariably run out of self-regulatory gas when trying to maintain that weight loss over the long term. (Spoiler alert: Unless, of course, they learn to apply minimum-effort, maximum-efficiency strategies for sustaining weight loss.)

These findings provide both diagnostic insight and a prescriptive takeaway. They show that the high rate of relapse among dieters is rooted in physiological mechanisms, not merely a return to old habits. The takeaway lesson is this: since our self-control energy is *not* unlimited, it needs to be managed like any other finite resource and should not be squandered. To succeed in the long term, we will need to develop and implement sustainable maintenance strategies that deploy self-control energy efficiently. This approach stands in sharp contrast to the so-called "knockout" (KO) solutions, which operate on the flawed premise that once target weight is reached, the journey is over… we're done.

The discouraging news, however, is that despite repeated failures and setbacks, many people still fail to fully learn this lesson. Which brings us to the second common miscalculation: *over*-estimating our capacity to learn from failure.

Failure to Learn from Failure

> *The definition of insanity is doing the same thing over and over and expecting different results.*
>
> Albert Einstein

As already noted, the dual blows of failing to attain desired weight loss goals and struggling to maintain even modest losses rarely prompt people to pause and reflect on the reasons behind their setbacks or to question their strategies. Instead, what do dieters typically do? Most often, they blame their challenges on not trying hard enough and resolve to try anew… but harder. Occasionally, the disappointments might induce a *tweak* in tactics—for example, switching from a diet X to the new KO diet-du-jour Y.

The all too familiar result? Many remain stuck in a seemingly vicious cycle of weight loss and regain: gaining weight → seeking a quick-fix → under performance and relapse. *Yo-Yo dieting* has become the colloquial term for the dreaded phenomenon (Figure 1.3).

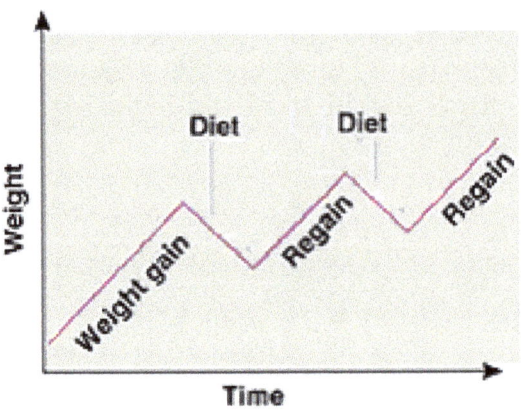

Figure 1.3. *Yo-Yo* Dieting

If you find yourself trapped in that exasperating pattern, you can take solace in knowing you are not alone.

Indeed, the collective anguish is inescapable. To see it—or feel it—all you have to do is glance at the tabloids stacked at the checkout counter of your local grocery store. You'll find many familiar faces on the cover pages baring personal tales of anguish and distress. There is a good chance, for example, you'll find Oprah Winfrey—the beloved TV talk show star who's had a long public battle with her weight—lamenting her latest upswing in jeans' size. Since the 1980s, after losing 67 pounds on a liquid diet and daily 6.5-mile runs, only to regain it all, she has candidly chronicled her roller-coaster journey with weight and food (Figure 1.4). (The latest—but surely not final—act: On March 18, 2024, she revealed in an ABC TV special that she is now combining the weight-loss medication Ozempic with hiking, regular workouts, and a healthy diet.)

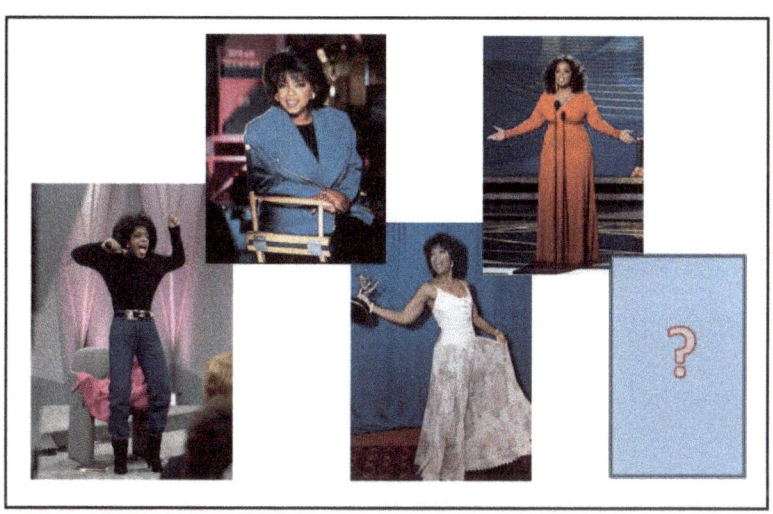

Figure 1.4
Snapshots from Oprah's roller-coaster ride

Oprah is but one of a growing cadre of female idols who have been speaking openly about their personal struggles with weight-loss-and-regain. Others include, (the late) Kirstie Alley, Maureen Marcia Brady McCormick, Janet Jackson, Kelly Clarkson... and the list goes on and on. While the celebrities' captivating travails grab the headlines, *Yo-Yo* dieting is not a price the rich and famous pay for the glamorous lifestyle. As an eloquent academic colleague of mine—who is neither rich nor glamorous—vividly put it: For many of us "chronic dieters," losing weight is akin to that cherry blossom in my backyard, a flower whose vivid beauty is accentuated by its brief existence!

Cherry blossoms aside, the record shows that the majority of dieters not only gain back most of the weight they lose, they often gain *more*! In one of the most comprehensive and rigorous investigations, researchers at the University of California at Los Angeles analyzed 31 long-term diet studies, and found that about two-thirds of regular dieters regained more weight within four or five years than they initially lost.[47]

While it's no surprise that failure to achieve and maintain a desired body weight rarely dissuades people from trying again and again, it is both surprising and unsettling that, despite the many travails, most never seem to learn enough to ultimately become long-term "successful losers." Why is that?

The academic answer: Learning from failure is not as straightforward as we might think, particularly when dealing with complex problems.[48] While true, the trite, abstract explanation is neither particularly helpful nor satisfying. Failure to learn from life's failures—not only with respect to body weight regulation, but generally—can be a serious handicap, and, thus deserves a fuller hearing. So, let us take a deeper dive to unpack the reasons behind what I am calling dieters' *learning disability*! And while at it, also try to understand how, despite the disability we often manage to compensate and carry on—not just in health, but across a wide spectrum of human decision-making.

Pursuing—and achieving—Goals… with and without Learning

Every day, we tackle numerous problems and make countless choices—whether at home, school, work, or on the road. Many of these choices are highly consequential, especially those related to our personal health. Yet, rarely do we stop to think about *how* we think. Perhaps we should.

It is widely understood that human behavior is purposeful, guided by our goals and objectives (e.g., the goal of losing weight). When we perceive a discrepancy between our current state and where we want to be—and assuming we have the will and the means—we take corrective actions to close that gap and move closer to our desired outcome (e.g., achieving a healthier body weight). And if we do not fully succeed, we may continue trying—probing, testing, accumulating experience. This iterative problem-solving process can unfold in markedly different ways—with or without *learning*—with important ramifications, Such as whether we ultimately succeed or fail and at what cost.

When tackling a problem or pursuing a goal, the choices we make and corrective actions we take are simultaneously governed by our *mental models* and the *outcome feedback* we receive from our actions.[49] These two cognitive elements are crucial in shaping a person's goal-seeking behavior and determining the ultimate success or failure of that behavior. Let's examine each of these factors in turn.

No one's mind holds an actual family, city, school, hospital, or business. Instead, all human decisions are guided by mental models—such as those of family dynamics, a city's layout, the hierarchy in a business, or how the body regulates weight. Mental models are deeply ingrained assumptions, generalizations, or even mental images we develop based on our past experiences, training, and instruction. These cognitive constructs are not simply repositories for past learning; they also shape how we interpret current situations and significantly influence how we act when pursuing our goals.[50]

Naturally, we like to think, and most us believe, that well-adjusted individuals possess relatively accurate mental models of themselves, their bodies, and their capacity to control important events in their lives. Unfortunately, this is not the case. And, what is more disturbing, most people are unaware of this situation.[51] A great deal of research in cognitive psychology has revealed that mental models are only simplified abstractions of the experienced world and are often incomplete, reflecting a world that is only partially understood.[52,53,54] (See sidebar.) No wonder, we often miss the mark—at least initially.

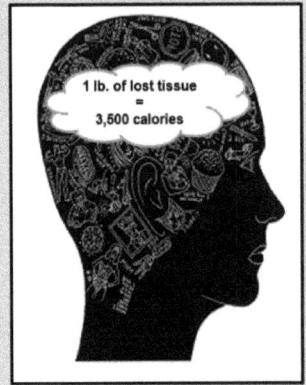

Mental Models
Can be simplistic... even inaccurate

1 lb. of lost tissue
=
3,500 calories

A widely held but inaccurate mental model about body weight regulation is that creating a weekly caloric deficit of 3,500 calories—whether through diet or exercise—leads to a loss of exactly one pound/week. The underlying assumptions being: 1) that a pound of lost tissue (no matter its composition) is worth 3,500 calories; and 2) that energy can be treated as though it were a single currency. Meaning, that cutting 3,500 calories from one's diet is *equivalent*—in terms of weight loss—to burning 3,500 extra calories through increased exercising.

Both of these model assumptions are incorrect, and the error matters. For instance, it can lead to overly optimistic predictions about treatment outcomes. Additionally, the misconception about diet and exercise equivalency often encourages people to underestimate the value of exercise, leading them to choose the easier, faster path of dietary restriction alone.

Yet, despite simplified, incomplete, or even inaccurate mental models, we often manage to make corrective adjustments and muddle our way toward achieving certain goals— including, at times, losing some weight. This is largely thanks to the *outcome feedback* we receive on our actions. The iterative problem-solving process of acting to achieve some goal → receiving feedback on the outcome → and making course corrections if needed (referred to in the literature as action-feedback-adjustment), can unfold in very different ways—with or without genuine learning—with significant consequences. The outcomes can determine not only whether we ultimately succeed or fail but also the costs involved.

First, let us see how this can work *without* learning.

In my university teaching, I've found that the clearest and most transparent analogy for goal seeking without real learning is an electromechanical one—the goal-seeking operation of your trusted home thermostat. The thermostat does its work by relying on sensors that provide its controller with continuous *outcome feedback* on what the actual status of a room's temperature is. Whenever a discrepancy between desired and actual temperatures is detected, the thermostat initiates corrective action—switching heating or cooling devices on or off—to bring room temperature back in line with our desired goal. The thermostat's monotonic routine of *action* → *outcome feedback* → *adjustment* provides an electromechanical analogy for the human mental model. As I'll explain below, this is the archetypal form of goal-seeking *without* learning—for both humans and machines—that works most of the time, though, *not* all of the time.

For instance, if one or more windows in the house develop a leak—perhaps due to cracked frames or deteriorating glazing—the most efficient solution to maintain the home's temperature would be to fix those leaks… and pronto. Alas, this is the kind of unscripted fix that the thermostat can never <u>learn</u> to implement. The thermostat's only recourse in this drafty-window situation is to keep doing what it has been programmed to do—rely on its temperature sensors' *outcome feedback* to cycle heating and cooling devices on and off as needed. While it may very well succeed in maintaining the desired temperature by working longer and harder, the cost to the homeowner will be a steep one—reflected in a hefty energy bill.

"Thermostating" is the text-book example to illustrate the limitations and costs of goal attainment without learning. Lest you may be wondering if such learning-free goal-seeking is limited to the realm of the electromechanical, in the next section I'll share a very *human* example—from yours truly!

Indeed, the thermostat-like monotonic *action* → *feedback* → *adjustment* routine is the customary, almost habitual, form of problem-solving that we often we rely on when pursing many of our goals. As when a dieter who fails to lose a desired amount of weight on diet X, then switches to a more aggressive diet Y, later to diet Z—modifying the intensity of caloric deprivation intensity but *not* her fundamental, possibly faulty, weight-energy calculus. (Hope you've read the sidebar above.) And ultimately achieving some satisfaction. This ingrained, almost instinctive inclination to tackle problems in a thermostat-like fashion—by working harder or longer, not differently— is neither unreasonable nor necessarily irrational.[55] Cognitively, it is an efficient, low-cost strategy that does not require us to reason anew in every situation. And even more pragmatically, it is often good enough to get the job done—for simple problems.

The potential pitfall: getting carried away and overplaying it.

As we shall see, on complex or non-routine decision tasks, monotonic problem-solving without learning is rarely effective. Sure, it may allow us to scratch and claw our way close to a goal, but more often than not it would get us there in an inefficient and costly fashion. And more importantly—as on weight loss endeavors—it is almost always a provisional, *temporary* fix.

As I illustrate with a personal story below, tackling complex problems—such as relating to human health and disease—calls for a more enlightened mode of problem-solving: goal-seeking with genuine learning. This involves two key steps: (1) recognizing that our current mental model—for instance, about weight and energy regulation—is not up to scratch; and (2) being open to incorporating new insights from experience, study, or guidance (such as from reading this book) to construct a more effective model for achieving our goals. We consider genuine learning to have occurred when a novel solution is ultimately produced and adopted.

Unlike the relatively straightforward and often automatic cycle of action → outcome feedback → adjustment, gaining a new conceptual understanding of a problem is neither easy nor automatic—and thus, not common. But it doesn't have to be elusive. While it may not be as routine or spontaneous, as I'll demonstrate throughout this book, it is *not* beyond our reach.

But first, as promised, I'll share a personal experience from a few years ago that demonstrates the mental "gear-shifting" between these two problem-solving modes as well as illustrate the important performance implications. Since this story isn't directly about weight loss, consider it optional reading—but I do believe you'll find it offers some interesting and relevant insights.

Difference between a Muddling-One's-Way Strategy and *Enlightenment:* A Personal Story

The story begins many years ago on the waters of San Francisco Bay, where I first learned to sail on a charming little sailboat I owned. Setting off from the marina along the city's waterfront, I would initially steer toward my chosen destination for the day—say to the Alcatraz lighthouse—trim the sails, and head out. Given the bay's powerful currents and gusty winds, it was wise to keep a close watch on the boat's path to catch any drift off course. On days when the tides were particularly strong, significant drifting was common, sometimes pushing me uncomfortably close to a navigational buoy or other hazards. (On one memorable day, I narrowly avoided a collision with Little Alcatraz, a partially submerged rock about 75 meters off the northwest coast of Alcatraz Island.) Whenever I noticed I was off course, my usual response was standard practice: correct my steering to offset the deviation (also referred to as the off-track error) and redirect the boat back toward my destination.

These corrections were rarely one-time KO fixes however. Each adjustment would temporarily get me back on track, but inevitably and before long, the currents would nudge me off track again. In effect, my approach became a repeating cycle: steering to destination→ drifting off course→detection of the deviation→and correction. Although we almost always reached our destination, my (fairly typical) steering strategy highlights how reliance on an action-and-adjustments routine can indeed get you to your goal—albeit at a high cost. In this case, my track to the destination was a *crooked*, inefficient course as clearly depicted in Figure 1.5.

Such a zigzagging-type progression to goal is a telltale of action-feedback-adjustment problem-solving. Whether in sailing, thermostating, or weight regulation. (Notice how my zigzagging course—if you look at it from the side—bears a striking similarity to the *Yo-Yo* dieting pattern depicted in Figure 1.3.)

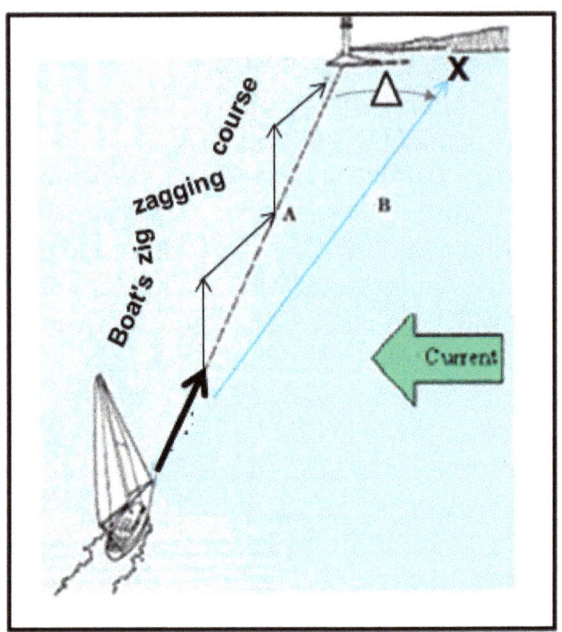

Figure 1.5: What course to the lighthouse?

Clearly, such a "crooked" course is <u>not</u> the fastest course to the lighthouse. There is a better way. Fortunately for me—and my crew—I eventually figured it out. (Full disclosure: I owe my "breakthrough" to a navigational article I came across in *Latitude 38*, a respected local sailing publication, which included all the necessary trigonometric calculations.) The trick to sailing the shortest non-zigzagging course to a desired destination in San Francisco Bay is to account for the current's estimated effect. This means steering the boat slightly *into the current*—towards point "X" in Figure 1.5—assuming the current is moving from right to left, and we are heading for the lighthouse. (Determining how much of an offset is needed, represented by Δ in the figure, required careful but straightforward navigational calculation.) Provided the current's strength was accurately estimated, the boat's heading toward "X" would only need to be set <u>once</u>. As the boat moves through the water, the current would gradually "eat" into the offset, slowly steering us toward the true goal—

the lighthouse. Instead of zigzagging, the boat would follow the most direct and efficient course to its destination.

Learning to work <u>with</u> the current, rather than fighting it, was a bona fide *Judo-esque* eureka moment for me. It planted the seed—years later—for what I am advocating here: that we need to work with our bodies' physiology, not against it, to effectively regulate body weight.

Before leaving the sailing metaphor behind and getting back to the business at hand—body weight regulation—I generalize below the insights gleaned from my sailing (mis)adventures:

- Despite crude and/or incomplete mental models, we are often able to muddle our way towards attaining many of our goals... thanks to the *outcome feedback* we receive on our actions.
- The *thermostat-esque* strategy works, but often only temporarily. And can be an inefficient (and crooked) path towards attaining our goals.
- Tackling complex problems effectively demands a more enlightened approach.
- Learning entails a *willingness* to question ingrained mental models and the *skill* to revise or enhance one's conceptual understanding of a task or problem, ultimately leading to the development of novel—and ideally more effective—solutions.

On a leisurely sail across the bay, the cost of sticking to a monotonic, learning-free strategy was a little delay and the inconvenience of back-and-forth tacking. However, in the case of *Yo-Yo* dieting and managing body weight, the consequences of being unwilling or unable to question and revise ingrained misconceptions—of which there are many, as we'll see—can be far more serious, with risks to both our health and well-being.

Ingrained Weight-Loss Misconceptions

Arguably, it is the mother of all misconceptions: that deeply entrenched—and highly consequential—belief that the task of maintaining a healthy body weight can be entrusted to the so-called "wisdom of our body." (The sidebar below delves into the appeal and underlying assumptions of this idea.) It's obviously very comforting to believe that the body's energy regulation system is wisely *symmetrical*, even-handedly defending against both weight loss and gain, while striving to maintain stability at a "normal" body weight. And surprise, surprise, it is also the implicit—and very convenient—premise of knock-out (KO) weight-loss strategies: that once we attain our target weight, we are done. The body's *symmetrical* weight regulation system would (wisely) keep us there.

If you believe that, please email me… I have a KO weight-loss strategy (and a bridge in Brooklyn) to sell you!

In reality, as briefly mentioned earlier and explored in greater detail in Chapter 3, the body's weight and energy regulation system is *asymmetric*—a system that favors over-consumption and strongly defends against negative energy balances and weight loss. Indeed, it is the mismatch between our body's asymmetric system of weight-energy regulation and our modern obesifying environment that explains why we are all at risk of weight-gain and relapse after weight loss. It also explains why knock-out strategies seldom deliver lasting results.

> ## *WISDOM OF THE BODY?*
>
> Throughout much of human history, humans have learned to instinctively regulate behavior in accordance with the body's signals: eat when hungry (when the body senses an energy deficit) and stop eating when feeling full (when energy depots are replenished). Given that obesity was never a common health problem, it is quite understandable that our ancestors instinctively believed in the body's "wisdom" to defend against both weight loss and weight gain while striving to maintain stability at some "normal" body weight. Even today, feeding behavior for many remains set on "cruise-control"—largely accomplished unconsciously and automatically, and requiring little deliberate effort. Unfortunately, this is an illusion—and a risky one—that may lull people into a false sense of invulnerability and seriously undermine obesity prevention.
>
> So, why was *ad libitum* feeding behavior OK for thousands of years... but is not anymore?
>
> Throughout much of human history, humans lived as hunter-gatherers in an environment where food was scarce and the next meal unpredictable. To help us succeed in a food-scarce environment, nature compensated and equipped us with an asymmetric regulatory system that favors over-consumption and strongly defends against negative energy balances. And it worked! It allowed our hunter-gatherer ancestors maintain their energy reserves at substantial enough levels to provide a buffer against prolonged periods of food shortages. The fact that obesity wasn't a realistic possibility for our ancestors was a result of the "fit" between this asymmetrical system—that drove them to eat voraciously when food was plentiful, and store the excess energy efficiently as a buffer against future food shortages—and their food-scarce environment.
>
> Today, we are not always so lucky. The same physiologic adaptations that kept us alive and in good form in a hunter-gatherer environment are resulting in a maladaptive response in our modern food-rich, activity-poor environment. Our pro-consumption physiological system is still intact, still encouraging us to overeat. And with constant access to an abundant supply of high-calorie, high-fat food and a sedentary lifestyle that has reduced our energy requirements, there is constant pressure on the system towards positive energy balance (and weight gain).
>
> (In Chapter 3, I explain how the asymmetry in human energy regulation works and in part II, I discuss strategies for achieving successful and sustainable weight loss despite it.)

This is just one of many enduring misconceptions that persist despite abundant counterevidence—and personal experiences of failures. (Another: the ubiquitous 3,500 kcal per pound rule, namely, that 3,500 kcal energy deficit per week causes a loss of one pound per week, two pounds in two weeks, and so on.) To be fair, this apparent "learning disability"—the inability to realize when our mental models are deficient—is not confined to weight loss and the overweight. As already noted, learning to use life's raw experiences (and occasional setbacks) to revise long-standing beliefs is hard and, therefore, uncommon.[56] A significant barrier to enlightenment—especially when dealing with a highly complex and relatively opaque system such as human physiology—is that the deficiencies in our mental models are often not readily apparent. In the case of dieting and body weight regulation, for example, there are many uncertainties—even on such basics as the precise caloric content of the foods we consume. Additionally, a range of confounding variables—such as travel, illness, medications, stress, exercise habits, and changes in smoking—can all impact body weight fluctuations. All of this means that there will be too many ways for people to explain away the mismatch between expectations—such as maintaining a stable weight after dieting—and actual results, leaving them feeling little need to question or revise their mental models—such as the magic number 3,500 kcal/lb.

Even when the evidence is clear enough to compel learning or a change in perspective, in situations like dieting and body weight management—where our self-esteem is at stake—we are naturally biased to interpret that evidence in a way that protects our self-image. For instance, rather than blaming our chosen strategy, on which we may have invested significant time, money, and effort, we may shift the blame to external factors like increased job stress, holiday celebrations, illness, and so on. And so, in situations marked by complexity, ambiguity and imperfect information, misconceptions often persist. And persist.

The price? Just as with my rookie sailing (mis)adventures, sticking to deficient weight-loss strategies *may* allow us to scratch and claw our way towards a target weight, but it will almost always be a brief cherry-blossom-like success... and zigzaggingly agonizing over the long-term.

We need to do better.

Indeed, when it comes to personal health, we must do better. For, unlike home heating or a leisurely sail on the bay, personal health is precisely the domain where failures are most consequential and where the stakes are the highest.

Research findings consistently confirm that weight-cycling—the hallmark of a thermostat-like, learning-free approach to weight management—poses significant risks to both physical health and emotional well-being. Beyond the emotional toll of repeated disappointment and lowered self-esteem, the physical consequences can be severe. Studies show that repeated cycles of weight loss and regain are associated with increased risks of chronic conditions, particularly coronary heart disease, and may even contribute to premature mortality.[57, 58]

Still, concerns about weight cycling should not be an excuse to resign ourselves to living with excess weight.

The Heavy Burden of Excess Weight

Please keep this in mind: even modest levels of excess body fat—just ten to twenty pounds above a healthy weight—can harm your health.[59] That's because body fat, which was once thought of as little more than an inert storage depot, is now understood to be a highly active metabolic organ. The hormones and chemical substances it releases can flood the body, damaging blood vessels, causing insulin resistance, and promoting cancer cell growth.[60] For example, one recent study found that individuals with a body mass index (BMI) over 30 were 1.7 times more likely to have heart disease, twice as likely to suffer from hypertension, and three times as likely to have diabetes compared to those of normal weight..[61] Another study examining cancer risk reported that excessively overweight men and women were three times more likely to develop kidney cancer, while obese post-menopausal women had up to a 50% higher risk of developing breast cancer compared to their non-obese counterparts.[62]

And then came COVID-19, which was like pouring gasoline on a smoldering fire!

Early in the pandemic, doctors noticed that people carrying excess weight were more susceptible to severe cases of COVID-19, more likely to require intensive care, and faced a higher risk of death.[63] These observations were soon backed by empirical research. One study found that individuals with obesity or overweight who contracted COVID-19 were more than twice as likely to be hospitalized and nearly 50% more likely to die from the virus. Another study, examining nearly 17,000 hospitalized COVID-19 patients in the United States, revealed that over 77% had excess weight or obesity.[64]

Since overweight and obesity often come with other health issues, researchers initially questioned whether excess fat itself contributed directly to severe COVID-19 outcomes. Now, years into the pandemic, a growing body of evidence indicates that it does, at least in some patients.

Research is also beginning to explain why. Experimental studies have shown that the coronavirus can directly infect fat cells, whose immune defenses appear limited and ineffective against the virus. In these cells, the virus can replicate and stage further attacks on the body. (The notion that adipose tissue could serve as a reservoir for pathogens isn't new; body fat is already known to harbor viruses like HIV and influenza.) [65] Additionally, abdominal obesity—which is more prevalent in men—can compress the diaphragm, lungs, and chest cavity, making it harder to breathe and to clear pneumonia or other respiratory infections.[66]

While COVID-19 may be the latest distress (SOS) signal, it's unlikely to be the last. As science marches ahead and the methods for studying disease become more sophisticated, we can expect the news about overweight and ill-health to grow even worse.[67]

It is why, I believe, fighting *smartly* to attain and maintain a healthy weight has never been more important.

Willpower alone is not Enough

> *Even the best intentions and strongest motivations are often not enough to help seriously overweight people lose a significant amount of weight and, more important, keep it off.*
> Jane E. Brody[68]

As I mentioned earlier, but it bears repeating: the fact that millions struggle to lose weight and maintain that loss—despite investing significant time, money, and effort—strongly suggests that the problem isn't a lack of *will*; it's a lack of *skill*. Specifically, it reflects limited public understanding of the body's energy regulation system and a failure to craft effective strategies to counterbalance its inherent asymmetries. It is a failure that leads many of us to expend (waste) too much effort battling our own body. It's similar, if I may harken back to my earlier boxing analogy, to a boxer throwing mostly wasteful punches at an opponent assuming a protected *rope-a-dope* stance (Figure 1.6). (The rope-a-dope is a boxing fighting technique perfected by the great Muhammad Ali, in which he would lean against the ropes of the boxing ring and draw non-injuring offensive punches, letting the opponent tire themselves out.)

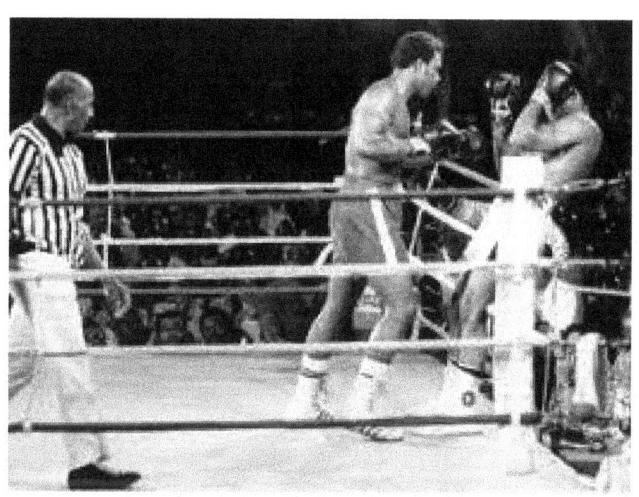

Figure 6
Muhammad Ali in a Rope-a-dope Stance

Wasting too much energy when trying to lose weight is similarly problematic because, as we will learn in Chapter 7, our self-regulatory capacity is a limited resource that—as previously emphasized—needs to be efficiently managed and must not be squandered. And that, too, requires *skill*.

So, remember, willpower alone is *not* enough. It rarely is for most worthy endeavors. Whether you are trying to ace an exam or lose weight, the two capacities—will and skill—are needed *together* to succeed. If either is lacking, the chance for success diminishes, regardless of how strong the other may be. It's like the simple multiplication equation "A x B" in basic algebra: if either factor is zero, the entire result is zero, no matter how high the other number might be. If the skill to devise effective and efficient interventions is lacking, for example, long-term success will elude us no matter the will and enthusiasm for change. Similarly, an absence of will to change renders any good solutions academic.

Given the time and money you've invested in acquiring and reading this book, I'm confident you already possess the necessary *will* to succeed. Hence, the focus in *Slim Samurai* is on building your weight and energy regulation *skill*. Specifically, the aim is to enhance your conceptual understanding—your mental model, if you will—of the body's weight and energy regulation system. This will empower you to develop effective weight-loss strategies tailored to your unique health needs and lifestyle preferences. More concretely, the book will guide you in devising *Judo-inspired*, high-leverage strategies that work in harmony with your body's inherent (asymmetric) physiological processes, rather than fighting against them.

And here is the good news: it can be done.

The best evidence that long-term weight-loss success is not a fantasy comes from the experiences of countless individuals who have participated—and continue to participate—in the National Weight Control Registry (NWCR).)[69] Founded in 1994 by Rena Wing of Brown Medical School and James O. Hill at the University of Colorado, the NWCR is the largest study of successful weight loss maintenance in the U.S. Its purpose is to track and learn from individuals who have succeeded in maintaining long-term weight loss. Today, the NWCR is managed by the Miriam Hospital's *Weight Control and Diabetes Research Center* in Providence, Rhode Island, and includes approximately 10,000 individuals who have lost weight and kept it off for an extended period.

The data from these "successful losers" clearly show that long-term weight loss is achievable through smart cognitive strategies that aim to override our innate biological instincts (though not necessarily the *Judo-inspired* methods I advocate here). The key takeaway: sustainable weight loss is undeniably possible... if approached *correctly*. The hard truth, though, is that there are no knock-outs! Achieving long-term success requires strategies that can be sustained for the long haul—not for a week, a month, or even a year, but possibly for a lifetime.

Metanoia

> *To achieve something you've never had, you must be willing to do something you've never done.*
> Thomas Jefferson

Albert Einstein once observed that the significant problems we face cannot be solved at the same level of thinking we were at when we created them. That we'd have to shift to a new level, a deeper level of thinking, to solve them. Going back in history even further, the Greeks had coined a wonderful word for the mental jumps to new ways of thinking and acting that we often need to make: *metanoia*. It means a fundamental shift of mind or, more literally, transcendence *(meta*—above or beyond, as in metaphysics) of mind (noia, from the root *nous,* of mind).[70]

It may be time for a *metanoic* jump in tackling the weight-loss project. In *Slim Samurai*, I argue for tackling body weight regulation by working with the body not against it. A novel—*Judo*-inspired—way of thinking.

The philosophical principles and foundational concepts of the *Judo way* are introduced in Chapter 2. At its core, Judo emphasizes the importance of first assessing one's opponent—gauging their strengths and weaknesses—before engaging. In this spirit, before diving into the *Judo*-inspired strategies of Part II, Chapter 3 will guide us in studying the intricacies of the human weight and energy regulation system. The aim is to deepen your understanding of how this complex physiological system functions—how processes like energy intake and expenditure are interconnected, how they influence one another, and how they are affected by the external environment. Understanding how and why the system behaves the way it does and what effects our interventions will or will not have is essential in identifying *leverage* points in the system and, thus, in devising appropriate interventions for change.

Chapter 2

The Judo Way

Eureka!

My judo epiphany came a few years back, while watching a young female judoka face off against a much taller, heavier male opponent. For over two minutes, she held her ground, skillfully using wily judo moves to absorb and redirect the force of his attacks, effectively neutralizing his strength advantage. Her opportunity to finish him off came two and a half minutes into the fight when her visibly tiring opponent lunged toward her. Instead of resisting, she drew him forward, using his own momentum to pull him across her hip, breaking his balance. With the big guy overextended and vulnerable, she lifted him—using her hip as fulcrum to gain *leverage*—twisted him and brought him crashing down at her feet. It was a stunning display of the aptly named *O goshi* throw (Figure 2.1). *O gosh* indeed!

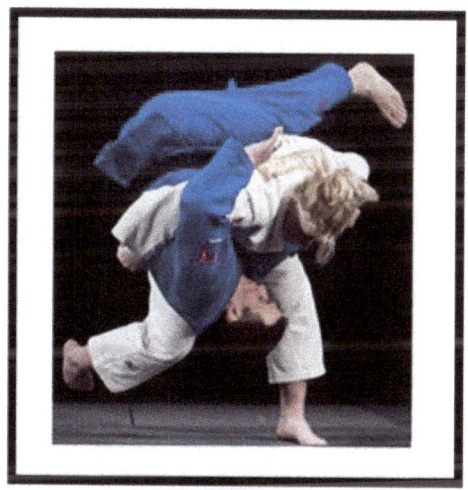

Figure 2.1: *O-goshi* throw

The young woman's execution of this classic judo throw—seemingly effortless yet strikingly effective—was a poignant demonstration of one of judo's core principles: *Seiryoku-Zenyo*, or "maximum efficiency, minimum effort." This guiding principle defines judo's distinctive approach, shaping how force is applied, resisted, or redirected with precision and economy, and serves as the foundation for its myriad attack and defense techniques.

Rather than countering an attack or a push with an opposing force of equal or greater magnitude—a losing proposition when facing a larger, stronger opponent—judo teaches the art of blending into the opponent's force and using their own strength and momentum against them. If the attacker pushes, you pull. If the attacker pulls, you push. This transfer of power, combined with a deep understanding of leverage, angles, and balance, enables smaller judokas to generate the favorable leverage needed to lift and throw much larger opponents with minimal exertion—just as I had witnessed.

Watching the young woman overcome her formidable opponent—with "maximum efficiency, minimum effort"—was a bona fide Eureka moment, one that would ultimately become the foundation for this book. I remember wondering, perhaps even musing: could the same efficient, opportunistic strategy of working *with*, not *against*, one's opposition provide dieters the leverage they need to succeed in the battle against weight gain?

The deeper I delved into judo's teachings and philosophical underpinnings, the more the idea resonated and seemed promising. Interestingly, the more I explored, the more confident I grew that my "hack" of the *Judo way* in service of personal health wouldn't have unsettled Judo's founder, Dr. Jigoro Kano. On the contrary, interjecting Judo principles into the global "battle of the bulge," might well have gratified him.

As I will elaborate below, Dr. Jigoro Kano always envisioned judo as more than just a martial art. Early on, he emphasized that judo's principles are universal and profound, urging his disciples to practice its precepts in their daily lives—beyond the *dojo*. The essence of the *Seiryoku-Zenyo* principle—making the most efficient use of one's mental and physical energy in the pursuit of goals—was something he tirelessly preached, reminding them that it applied broadly to their everyday lives, no matter the endeavor.

He was, of course, correct.

Indeed, many of us instinctively apply— or at least attempt to apply— his philosophy when we strive to use our limited resources, such as time and money, *efficiently* in both our personal and professional lives. For example, we do this when hunting for a good deal while shopping or researching the quickest route when driving to a destination. In competitive sports, elite athletes—whether long-distance runners, swimmers, tennis players, or others—are trained to use physical energy efficiently in order to outlast the competition. Similarly, businesspeople and even politicians aim to optimize the expenditure of effort and resources—whether for advertising campaigns or upgrading city infrastructure—to get the most "bang for the buck."

Surprisingly, however, the "maximum efficiency – minimum effort" ethos has not extended to the management and regulation of personal health. This is a missed opportunity—a shortcoming we aim to address and rectify in this book.

But first, a brief overview of the origins of judo.

A Brief History… and Overview of Judo's Philosophical Underpinnings

> *The pine fought the storm and broke. The willow yielded to the wind and snow and did not break. Practice Jiu-Jitsu in just this way.*
>
> 7   Jigoro Ka*no*

Judo was created by Dr. Jigoro Kano in the 1880s when he sought to synthesize several *Jujitsu* styles that were in practice at the time—the traditional unarmed combat arts of the professional samurai warrior class. His primary goal was to preserve these ancient and cherished arts, which he, along with many others, feared were at risk of fading away after Japan overthrew feudalism and dissolved the samurai class in 1877. Kano viewed the various *Jujutsu* styles of the time as disconnected sets of ingenious "tricks and devices" designed for professional samurai, and sought to unify them around a core set of principles, making them more accessible and safer for the "common man."

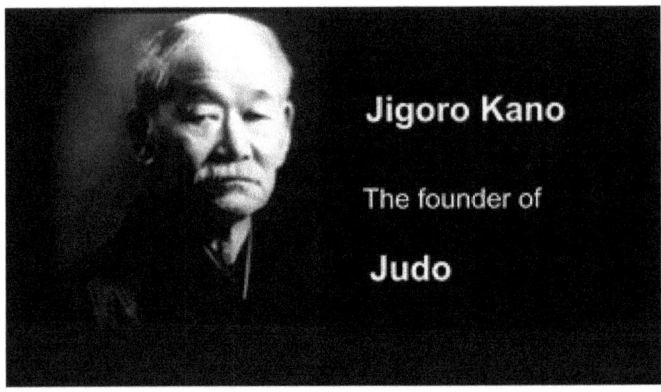

Figure 2.2 The father of judo

    Various records and accounts have been passed down through the ages regarding the true meaning of *Jujitsu*. The name is believed to be derived from the expression *ju yoku go o seisu*, which translates to "softness controls hardness." To Kano, the term represented a core principle that he not only embraced but would faithfully infuse into his new discipline, aptly named the *Judo*. The word *Judo* shares the same root ideogram as *Jujutsu*: the *"jū,"* which can mean "gentleness," "softness," "suppleness," and even "easy," depending on the context, and the *"do"* meaning "way." Hence, *Judo* is the soft or gentle way.
    In conceiving his new interpretation of martial art, Kano discarded or adapted those *Jujutsu* techniques that relied solely on superior strength or directly opposing an opponent's force, favoring techniques that involved blending with and redirecting the opponent's force. He studied and applied scientific principles related to mechanical leverage, angles of force (or "vectors"), and balance (center of gravity) to develop innovative combat techniques that provided superior leverage for maximum efficiency. What emerged was a repertoire of elegant and efficient tactics

for both attack and defense, requiring minimal exertion and no need for massive strength—a nod to the "common man."

The principle of maximum efficiency – minimum effort will be particularly relevant to us in this book. At its core, it embodies an "economy of means" concept that's easy to agree with—regardless of the endeavor—though not always easy to pull off. In Judo, this principle is realized through mastery of leverage—the leverage gained by working with, not against, an opponent's force, and using their power and momentum to augment one's own, thereby generating even more force. In simple terms, it works like this: If, for instance, a larger male opponent has a strength of six and a smaller female judoka has a strength of four, and they both push against each other with all their might, her four will inevitably lose to his six. However, if she pulls while he pushes, she harnesses the combined force of both bodies—ten units in total—and greatly improves her chances of prevailing.

To fully harness and further amplify the leverage gained through the transfer of an opponent's power and momentum (and secure the win), the judoka must also adopt proper positioning and throw mechanics. The stance, movement, and execution of throws in Judo are meticulously choreographed and, as mentioned earlier, are based on an intensive study of balance (center of gravity), angles of force (or "vectors"), and the mechanics of throws and movements. For example, using the hip as fulcrum to gain *leverage* when lifting a heavier opponent in the *O goshi* throw. This is why Judo is widely regarded as the most *scientific* of all martial arts.

Teaching how to bring an opponent down onto the mat was not Kano's sole or paramount goal however.

From the very beginning, his vision was more ambitious than merely creating a new combat art. An educator of great intelligence, compassion, and foresight, Dr. Kano infused his teachings with the ethics and moral code of *Bushido*—the samurai code of honor, courage, loyalty and justice. From his writings and teachings, it is clear that he deeply believed a martial art should not only strengthen the body and provide self-defense skills, but also stimulate the mind and nourish the spirit. Martial arts, he felt, must serve as a guiding force in the perfection of human character; otherwise, they would produce experts in combat without conscience—unrestrained and lacking the principles needed to guide proper behavior.

He wanted his art to influence society, and help his students grow as human beings. It was to this end that he founded his school—the *Kodokan*—in 1882.

What was both interesting and novel about the *Kodokan*, is the focus on teaching broader principles as opposed to just technique. While the primary goal of training in traditional *Jujitsu* was to learn methods for fending off attacks, Jigoro Kano was espousing something far more profound. Specifically, he emphasized the teaching of mental and physical strategies for using one's energy most effectively to achieve any goal—no matter the pursuit. He believed this was the ultimate purpose of studying human activity.

Nevertheless, fulfilling Kano's ambitious vision was predicated upon Judo's blossoming <u>as a sport</u>. Lucky for us, blossoming it did.

At its birthplace, Judo quickly gained popularity, and by the turn of the twentieth century, it had become Japan's dominant form of martial art. Not long after, it began spreading rapidly across the globe. The culmination of Judo's growth came in 1964 when it was included in the Olympics. Today, Judo sends more competitors to the Olympics from a wider range of countries than any other sport. Judo's excellent safety record has no doubt contributed to its broad appeal across cultures, genders, and generations. (It boasts the lowest injury rate of any combat martial art and one of the lowest injury rates of any sport.) According to the American College of Sports Medicine, Judo is also the safest contact sport for children. This is an undeniable testament to its "gentle way"!

In the U.S., one of the early and most famous proponents of Judo was President Teddy Roosevelt (1901-1909), who took Judo lessons while in the White House and earned a brown belt. Yet, despite the presidential cachet, Judo never managed to gain widespread popularity in America. Even today, it remains overshadowed by the rise of striking arts like karate, which gained mass attention through figures like Bruce Lee and the TV show *Kung Fu*. Perhaps it is because Americans have a tendency to seek quick results—and a well-placed punch or kick is a much quicker way to defend oneself. This cultural dynamic, I suspect, mirrors the widespread appeal of instant gratification in other areas, most notably fast food—a phenomenon linked to obesity, which we will explore in later chapters. (In the case of fast-food, the public seems to have unconsciously accepted the deterioration of their diet as a trade-off for convenience and time.) Similarly, in the case of Judo, the preference for a quick knockout may have overshadowed other qualities like safety, efficiency, and leverage.

Nevertheless, Dr. Kano's vision for the widespread cultural diffusion of Judo's principles—beyond just combat sport—did indeed come to fruition, even in the U.S.!

Beyond Combat... *Judo* as a Way of Life

> *Judo is not what many people believe it to be. For one thing, Judo is not just learning how to fight; it is learning how to live. I have emphasized that the basic meaning (philosophy) of judo is broader... it is universal and profound. The judo philosophy—of how to make the best use of one's mental and physical energy in order to achieve one's goals—applies across the spectrum of human activity.*
>
> The Teachings of Jigoro Kano

Judo's efficacy as a fighting skill and its reputation as a dominant martial art are well earned, with its techniques famously proving superior in widely publicized tournaments against other forms of *Jujitsu*. Yet, Jigoro Kano's true genius lay in his understanding that success in combat sports required not only ingenuity and the skillful use of various physical "tricks and devices." He saw that it was also about training the mind in essential ways—ways that extend beyond the mat and benefit life more broadly. This belief drove Kano's lifelong advocacy for martial arts as a means—not merely for self-defense—but as a guiding force in the cultivation of human character.

As in the quotation above, Kano emphasized the profound and universal appeal of Judo's core principles—chief among them *ju yoku go o seisu* (softness controls hardness) and *seiryoku zenyo* (maximum efficiency, minimum effort)—and he passionately espoused their value across all aspects of human behavior. It was his sincere hope that, through a thoughtful study of his writings, readers would come to appreciate the spirit of Judo and strive to live by its principles. He believed this would ultimately contribute to the betterment of society.

Kano's ambitions were not mere wishful thinking.

From the outset, in establishing Kodokan Judo, he organized it into three parts: its practice as a fighting method (martial art), as a method of physical training (physical education), and as a means of cultivating the mind, developing intellect and morals, and applying Judo's principles to everyday life. By structuring Judo in this way, Kano aimed to ensure that it would not be viewed merely as another martial art but embraced as a richer, more complex philosophical framework—a universal set of principles to be applied across all facets of human activity.

It may have taken longer than Kano anticipated, but today his vision has indeed been validated.

More than a century since the founding of Kodokan Judo, it has evolved into something far greater than a fighting art practiced at the *dojo*. The spirit of Judo has been embraced by politicians, business leaders, sociologists, and educators alike. Numerous books and articles espouse Judo's principles as applicable not only to physical education but also to intellectual training, management, social interaction, and even politics. Below is a sampling of book titles from *Amazon* and scholarly articles from *Google Scholar* that highlight the breadth of Judo's diffusion:

- *The Judo Strategy in Leadership*
- *Judo Management: Applying the Philosophy of Judo in Times of Great Uncertainty*
- *Judo Business Strategy: Turning Competitors' Strengths to one's Advantage*
- *Career Judo: The Martial Art for the Mindful Career*
- *Emotional Judo: Communication Skills to Handle Difficult Conversations and Boost Emotional Intelligence*
- *Verbal Judo: The Gentle Art of Persuasion*
- *The Public Opinion Judo-Throw: A Strategic Theory of Insurgent Propaganda and Political Violence*
- *Russian Judo: Putin's Diplomacy on the World Tatami Mat*

This list underscores the extensive reach of Kano's vision and the enduring influence of Judo's principles across diverse fields.

Conspicuously missing, however, is an application in personal health management—a lamentable oversight. For nowhere is the efficient use of energy more essential, and potentially more rewarding, than in managing personal health and well-being. Indeed, I submit, health is precisely the arena where inefficiencies—particularly in dealing with chronic or long-term conditions—can be most detrimental, with stakes at their highest.

One of my aims in this book is to illustrate the feasibility and utility of adopting the judoka's soft, efficient techniques—such as working with, rather than against, resistance—in managing personal health, and more specifically, in regulating body weight and energy. But before we turn to Judo-inspired strategies for weight management in Part II... first a *tsukuri*!

Because...

We Can't Manage What We Don't Understand

In Judo, every attack (*kake*) must be preceded by a *tsukuri* (preparatory action). This means preparing oneself (*jibun-no-tsukuri*) both physically and intellectually. In a combat setting, physical preparation involves positioning oneself in the most favorable posture to execute a defense or attack with maximum efficiency and minimal effort. But even before stepping into the arena to face an opponent, intellectual preparation is required. Judo teaches the importance of studying one's opponent to determine the most effective (and efficient) way to defend or attack.

Before we can execute an *O-goshi* on body fat, that's exactly what we will do next!

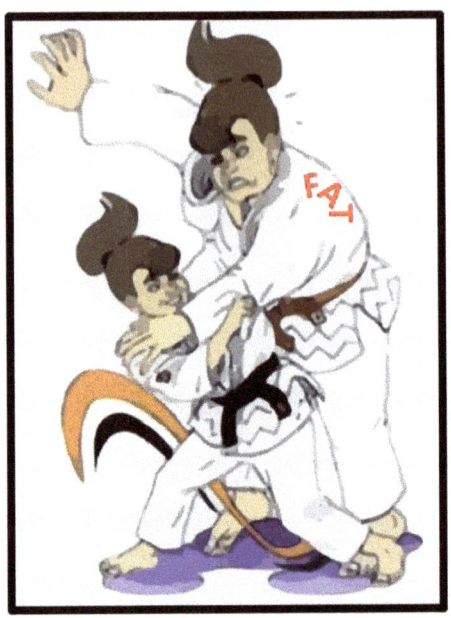

Figure 2.3: ***O-goshi*** <u>your</u> fat!

In Chapter 3—our *tsukuri* chapter, if you will—we "go to school" on the human weight and energy regulation system. The goal is to gain a deeper understanding of how this complex system works, how its processes (such as energy consumption and expenditure in the case of weight regulation) are interconnected, and how they influence one another and are affected by the system's external environment. Understanding how and why the system behaves the way it does, and what effects our actions will or will not have, is crucial for identifying *leverage* points in the system and, ultimately, for devising effective interventions for change (which we will explore in Part II).

Chapter 3

Tsukuri
Because we can't Manage what we don't Understand

People spend a lot of money, time and effort trying to defeat nature, rather than trying to understand how and why it works the way it does.
                                     Robert Mondavi, Winemaker

As you're reading this book, you're not consciously working to control your body's core temperature, are you?

Of course not. Like all animals, humans have evolved to rely on—and trust—our bodies' self-regulatory mechanisms to handle many essential functions from maintaining core temperature and balancing blood pressure to regulating blood glucose and more. Historically, this trust extended to managing our body's energy reserves.

As explained in the Prologue, for most of human history, people instinctively relied on their bodies' signals to regulate feeding behavior: eat when hungry—when the body signals an energy deficit—and stop eating when feeling full—when the body signals that energy stores are replenished. And for eons, this arrangement worked pretty well, keeping us alive and in reasonably good shape. Until now!

Five decades into the obesity epidemic, it's becoming increasingly clear that the long-standing assumption—that the body's weight and energy regulation system is "wisely" *symmetrical*, evenhandedly resisting both weight gain and loss to maintain stability at an ideal weight—is a fundamental misconception, and a risky one at that. In reality, as I mentioned earlier, humans are endowed with a weight-regulation system that is slightly *asymmetrical*.

As we'll learn in this chapter—an insight that will prove crucial for long-term weight maintenance—it only takes a slight degree of asymmetry to trigger weight gain in today's food-rich, activity-poor environment. Gains usually accumulate gradually, but over time they add up. Research shows that most people tend to gain weight at the slow rate of just a few pounds per year, underscoring that weight gain results from a remarkably small but persistent energy imbalance over an extended period. (For a typical adult with a daily intake of 2,000 to 2,500 kcal, this imbalance amounts to only about a 4 to 5 percent shift in total daily energy.)

To fully understand why the body's slightly asymmetric weight and energy regulation system, which kept us in good shape for thousands of years, is failing us now, we need to look back—way back—into our evolutionary history. An anthropological perspective reveals that the global obesity epidemic, particularly in Western cultures, is the result of a relatively recent mismatch between the modern living environment and a human physiology shaped by our evolutionary past. This mismatch began to take root when our ancestors shifted from a food-foraging lifestyle to food production thousands of years ago, but it didn't truly accelerate until the modern era, and with a vengeance in the second half of the 20th century.

Let me explain.

"Civilization is but a filmy fringe on the history of man"

By this phrase, the Canadian physician and historian William Osler meant that the past few millennia of human civilization represent only a tiny fraction of the time since our human ancestors first appeared on earth.[71] Archaeological data suggest that it was not until approximately 12,000 years ago that some human groups began shifting from a food-foraging lifestyle to one of food production. This shift was driven primarily by ecological pressures from population growth and food scarcities. It would prove momentous, as this relatively recent economic transformation ultimately enabled the evolution of complex societies and civilization itself.[72]

For hundreds of thousands of years before this "filmy fringe on our history," humans lived as hunter-gatherers, relying for nourishment on available game and on whatever fruits, nuts, berries, roots, leaves, and other vegetable matter was available.[73] While their diet was qualitatively adequate, food was often scarce and the next meal unpredictable, with starvation a constant threat in most prehistoric societies.[74]

Our understanding of life in ancient hunter-gatherer societies is based not only on the abundant archaeological evidence that we've accumulated, but also on the anthropologic study of *contemporary* hunter-gatherer populations. In what would surely qualify as a *Believe It or Not* story, there are still, at the dawn of the 21st century, some non-industrial societies that serve as "good approximations" of late Stone Age humans from about 20,000 years ago. Not just one or two, but a hundred or more.

Unsurprisingly, these societies have been the focus of intensive anthropological study. A cross-cultural ethnographic survey of over a hundred such societies found seasonal food shortages common across all of them—the same pattern revealed by archaeological studies of prehistoric hunter-gatherer skeletal remains. About half of these societies experience food shortages annually or more frequently, and in nearly a third of them, these shortages reach "severe" levels, approaching starvation.[75]

That's the bad news. The good news, however, is that these "best approximation" surrogates for our human ancestors exhibit slow population growth, enjoy high-quality (if not always high-*quantity*) diets, maintain high levels of physical fitness, and are generally healthy. In fact, they are healthier than many third-world populations currently undergoing economic modernization or westernization.[76]

That's no accident!

The interaction between a species—any species—and its food supply is one of the most important forces influencing biological adaptation and cultural evolution.[77] Because humanity's survival has historically been challenged by food scarcity, not abundance, the human body has evolved multiple redundant physiological systems to actively defend against this threat.[78] (Understanding these "multiple redundant physiological systems" and how they work is our task in this chapter.) And it has succeeded.

In the hunter-gatherer mode of existence, where a high level of physical activity was required for daily subsistence and the food supply was inconsistent, the challenge to the body energy-control system was to provide a strong drive to eat to keep pace with energy expenditure and to rest when physical exertion was not required.[79] And because starvation was not only real, but also a periodic threat, the greatest survival rates were among those who ate voraciously when food was plentiful and efficiently stored the excess energy as a buffer against future shortages.[80] Such individuals built up stores of fat that increased their survival prospects during famines, and they passed on these traits to their progeny, who, similarly, were more likely to survive. For the females—whose reproductive fitness depended on their ability to withstand the nutritional demands of pregnancy and lactation—greater energy reserves provided a selective advantage over their lean counterparts in withstanding the stress of food shortage, not only for themselves but for their fetuses and nursing children.[81]

Our taste buds are also deeply rooted in our evolutionary past. Thousands of years ago, when humans hunted wild game and gathered wild plants, their primary food sources contained limited amounts of sugar, fat, and salt. Yet, because these nutrients are essential to the body's proper functioning, it was beneficial for early humans to consume as much of them as they could find. To meet these dietary needs, evolution equipped us with a strong, nearly insatiable appetite for fat, salt, and sugar, encouraging us to seek out these foods. Over generations, these powerful taste preferences have been genetically passed down to us—and served us well—until now.

> Fatty foods helped our ancestors weather food shortages. Salt helped them maintain an appropriate water balance in their cells, helping avoid dehydration. Sugar and the sweetness associated with it helped them distinguish edible berries from poisonous ones. By giving us the taste for fat, sugar, and salt, our genetics led us to prefer the foods that were most likely to keep us alive. It also led us to want to eat a wide variety of foods. The more types of foods we could eat, the more we were likely to consume the wide range of unknown nutrients we needed. Our natural inclination for variety made sure we got enough of these

nutrients without us needing to know the difference between Vitamin C, riboflavin, and a complex carbohydrate.[82]

These now hardwired physiological mechanisms that regulate both the quantity and quality of our energy intake—favoring caloric overconsumption—are complemented on the energy-output side of the energy equation by homeostatic adaptations that regulate energy expenditure. Together, they provide a robust, double-barreled defense of the body's *energy reserves*. (As we'll see, this regulation of energy output is primarily achieved by adjusting the body's metabolic rate, for instance, lowering it in response to a negative energy balance or to conserve energy when physical activity is not required, such as after the day's hunt is over.[83])

In this evolutionary context, the usual range of human metabolic variation would have produced many individuals with a predisposition to become fat, but chronic food scarcity and vigorous physical exertion ensured that they never would.[84] Skeletal remains indicate that our human ancestors were typically leaner and more muscular than we are today. And studies of contemporary hunter-gatherer populations are consistent with this. For example, studies of the !Kung San tribe in the Kalahari Desert show them to be lean, with skin fold thicknesses approximately half those of age-matched North Americans and suffering no obesity problem.[85,86]

This suggests that, despite seasonal fluctuations in food availability and a mode of existence characterized by vigorous physical exertion, the caloric intake and output of our hunter-gatherer ancestors were balanced over time.[87] Eating whatever animals they could kill or scavenge and whatever fruit and vegetable matter they could take from plants, early humans kept enough fat stores to make it through the occasional lean times, but not so much that it slowed them down significantly.[88]

These findings provide an interesting insight: the long-term energy balance for our hunter-gatherer ancestors did not arise from a symmetric regulatory process or a stable environment, but from an *asymmetric* process that compensated for their unstable, food-scarce surroundings.

In the remainder of this chapter, you'll learn *how* asymmetry manifests in our 21st-century physiology. Understanding this is crucial if we are to identify the leverage points in the system and figure out how to work with it, not against it. But before we delve into that, I'll explain how our hunter-gatherer ancestors managed to achieve long-term energy balance despite environmental imbalance—and why this "evolutionary trick" is misfiring today.

Snatching Physiologic Balance from the Jaws of Environmental Imbalance

To maintain long-term stability in weight and energy reserves, nature evolved an energy regulatory system that does *not* aim for balance per se (i.e., energy in = energy out). Instead, to compensate for the unstable boom-and-bust food environment and achieve long-term stability, nature equipped us with an asymmetric regulatory system slightly tilted toward overconsumption, favoring a positive energy balance. "Fighting" external asymmetry with internal asymmetry is like fighting fire with fire—or, more abstractly, obtaining a *positive* result in arithmetic by multiplying two negative numbers.

Such "Judo-esque" adaptations—working with the environment not against it—are, it turns out, not uncommon in nature. Organisms, both simple and complex adapt to external stresses by evolving internal asymmetric structures and processes that cleverly compensate for, and even exploit, rather than fight their environmental challenges.[89] For example, trees growing in dense forests often experience asymmetrical sunlight availability due to the presence of neighboring trees. To compensate, trees can exhibit asymmetric growth patterns. For example, developing larger branches or leaves on one side, to reach out and capture more sunlight. This adaptation allows them to maximize their photosynthetic efficiency in low-light conditions and thrive in shaded environments.

Trees in dense forests and hunter-gatherer populations in food-scarce environments are two distinct examples of how very different types of organisms— whether animal or plant—can achieve stable equilibrium by "cleverly" evolving internal asymmetric mechanisms that compensate for the asymmetries in their external environments.

In the case of human energy regulation, the slightly asymmetric energy-regulation system worked effectively—and as intended—for thousands of years. The simplified diagram below (Figure 3.1) aims to illustrate graphically how this asymmetric system would have compensated for the short-term fluctuations in food availability and maintained long-term stability. During times of abundance, our asymmetric energy regulation system meant that we had a built-in drive to overeat to build up our fat reserves—as in point "A" (A for abundance). Given the chronic boom-bust cycles in food availability, these fat stores would be called upon every two to three years during periods of famine or food scarcity. During these times, body weight would drop, as illustrated at point "S" (S for starvation), but not for long and typically without adverse effects, thanks to the built-up fat reserves. And as good times eventually returned, body weight and energy reserves would rebound.

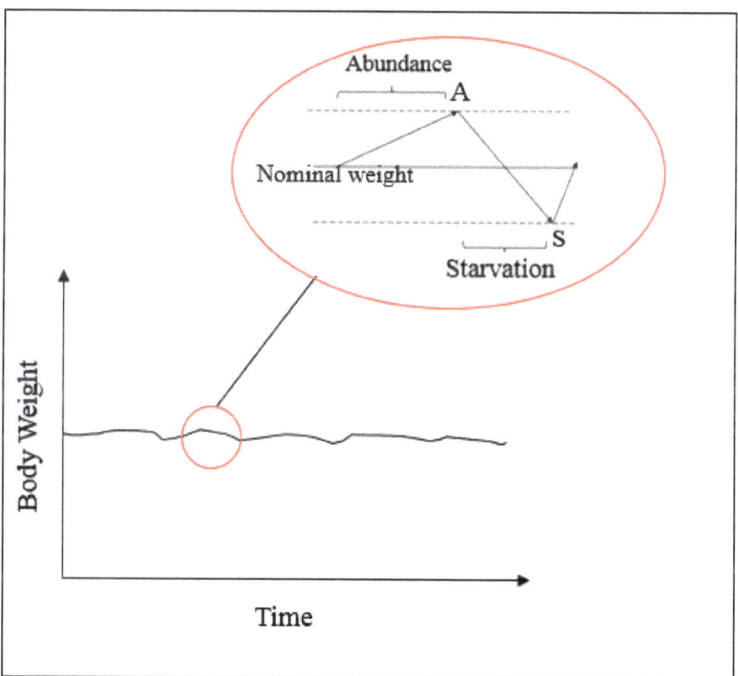

Figure 3.1 Body weight fluctuates seasonally, but is stable long-term

But could a *symmetric* system have worked as well? While it may seem counterintuitive, in a chronic boom-and-bust food environment, a *symmetrical* energy regulation system—one that defends *equally* against both weight loss and gain while striving to maintain stability at a "normal" body weight—would likely have led to extinction. How so?

The shortcoming of a symmetric system in a fluctuating food environment is that it does not provide an upside when food is plentiful to balance the downside when food is scarce. During food shortages weight would fall below "target"—that's the downside—while during periods of food abundance energy stores would only return to the target level without exceeding it, providing no upside to balance the downside. The inevitable result: weight will fluctuate within a range below the nominal level ... *not* around it. Over time, this means the average weight trends below target (Figure 3.2). The likely outcomes: frailty, disease, and possibly even extinction.

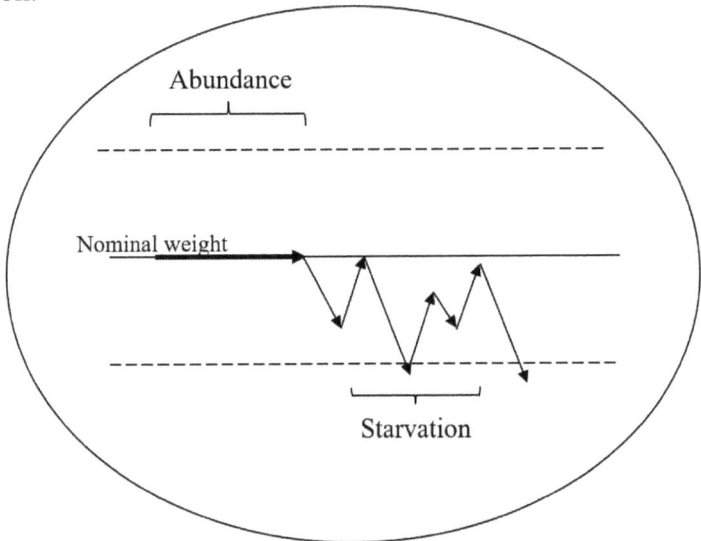

Figure 3.2. With *symmetric* energy regulation, body weight fluctuates below nominal

Professor Sam Savage of Stanford University offers an insightful analogy that illustrates how a symmetric model would likewise lead to bankruptcy (or "cash starvation") in a business context.[90] Imagine an entrepreneur planning to build a manufacturing facility for a new product.

After conducting a thorough market analysis, she estimates an average annual demand of 100,000 units. Further analysis of construction and operating costs suggests that a facility with a capacity of 100,000 units would yield a healthy $10 million annual profit.

What happens if, after going ahead with the plan, the demand does average 100,000 units but fluctuates significantly, ranging between 50,000 units ("famine" market conditions) and 150,000 units ("feast" market conditions)? Intuitively, most would expect profits to still average out to $10 million, with lower profits in some years balanced by higher profits in others. But that's not the case. Lower-than-average demand means profits fall below the target—there's the downside. Yet, when demand exceeds 100,000 units, the plant's capacity limits profits to $10 million, with no upside to offset the downside. The result: an average profit much lower than the "target," potentially leading to bankruptcy (or extinction).

(For the interested reader, this dynamic of fluctuating resources and survival has been explored in a multi-year computer simulation analyzing the interaction between food availability and hunter-gatherer survivability. This study, conducted by the author, is detailed in an academic paper titled *Eureka... Insights into Human Energy and Weight Regulation from Simple—Bathtub-like—Models*, which examines seasonal variation in food availability and survival strategies of the Hiwi hunter-gatherers in southwestern Venezuela.[91])

So, while we can say we're here today because our asymmetric system effectively compensated for a cyclical, unstable food environment over millennia, the recent upward trend in population weight suggests that this delicate equilibrium has been broken.

Flipping the Script... and Breaking the Balance

It's important to emphasize that successful evolutionary adaptations—where "balance is snatched from the jaws of imbalance"—are not absolute nor necessarily permanent successes since they are *relative* to the environment they arise within. For both people and trees, a happy equilibrium state is a dynamic state, adapted to specific conditions rather than absolute stability. So, if the environment shifts, as ours has rapidly in recent years, there's every reason to suspect that an adaptation once advantageous may lose its effectiveness—leading to imbalance and, ultimately, disequilibrium. (In physics, this phenomenon is known as *symmetry breaking*, where a previously balanced system tips out of equilibrium under new pressures.)

Devising internal asymmetric adaptations to manage external environmental challenges or imbalances can, thus, be both clever and effective—but it comes at a cost: inherent vulnerability. That's because if the environment changes, this carefully balanced "deal" is disrupted, and the internal asymmetric "solutions" that were once functional can become dysfunctional. In nature, this isn't often an issue, as environmental changes are typically slow, allowing most systems to re-adapt. Such disruptions simply exert pressure for new, adaptive designs. Indeed, this continuous cycle of change and adaptation drives evolution itself. While nature often seeks and achieves equilibrium, the world's dynamic texture is largely shaped by mechanisms of symmetry breaking!

But this re-adaptation process depends on synchronicity. When the pace of environmental change is faster than a system's capacity to adapt, problems arise as re-adaptation lags behind. This is precisely what we're seeing with human energy regulation. The tempo of human-made cultural and socioeconomic shifts has outpaced nature's slower rhythm of biological adaptation. Evolution in biology is a gradual process, with long lags between environmental changes and full evolutionary adaptation—a timeline that often spans many generations. Indeed, our current physiology reflects incremental adaptations extending millions of years into the past. In contrast, cultural and socioeconomic transformations have been swift, with dramatic shifts occurring within mere decades. This substantial difference in tempo has effectively thrown the once well-synchronized "biology-behavior-environment" dance out of step.

> **When Evolution Lags: The Fate of the Woolly Mammoth**
>
>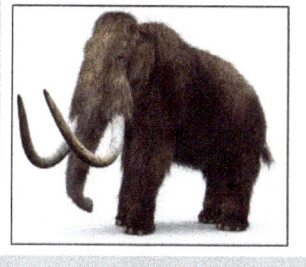
>
> While rare, this discordance can also occur in other species, perhaps due to uniquely slow-adapting genetic architectures. Take the woolly mammoths, for example: during the Ice Age, they adapted to frigid climates with thick fur and layers of insulating fat, traits that allowed them to flourish in icy grasslands. However, as the ice retreated and grasslands transitioned into dense forests, these large herbivores, adapted for open spaces, couldn't adjust quickly enough to the changing habitat. Their inability to navigate and thrive in forested areas led to diminished food resources, ultimately contributing to their extinction.

In the remainder of this section, I'll explain how rapid socioeconomic transformations have impacted both sides of the energy balance equation—energy intake (what we eat) and energy expenditure (how we use energy in work and play)—ultimately disrupting our longstanding adaptation to environmental conditions. To understand these changes, we'll need to examine both sides of the equation, as body weight depends on the relationship between the two. Like all systems, whether technological or biological, the human body obeys the laws of thermodynamics, including the fundamental principle of energy conservation: when energy intake and expenditure are balanced, weight remains stable. While a net excess in energy—whether from increased intake or reduced expenditure—must lead to weight gain.

How Energy *Input* Changed

As discussed earlier, for over 90 percent of our existence as a species, humans lived as hunter-gatherers, foraging for food. This way of life began to fundamentally change around 12,000 years ago when ecological pressures from population growth and food scarcities drove a shift from foraging to food production through farming.[92] This relatively recent transformation laid the foundation for the development of complex societies and, ultimately, civilization itself.[93]

Unfortunately, it also set the stage for the rise of obesity.

> (Indeed), obesity seems not to have appeared until after the development of agriculture and never to have affected more than a small percentage of any population until recently, when industrialized economies have created a luxurious living environment unlike anything ever seen before.[94]

The advent of farming enabled the production of a reliable food surplus, though early productivity was modest and food production was labor-intensive. This began to change significantly in the late eighteenth century with industrialization, which mechanized food production and greatly increased agricultural efficiency. Over the past century, advancements in mechanization, coupled with the growing use of chemical inputs—such as pesticides, fertilizers, veterinary drugs, and feed additives—led to massive economies of scale and a dramatic decline in food prices.

> Agriculture in developed countries has undergone startling change in the past 100 years. Vastly increased crop yields; reduced price of production; irrigation of previously unusable land; genetic engineering; and widespread use of fertilizers, pesticides, and antibiotics have transformed the basic economics of food.[95]

For example, in the United States, the share of average household income spent on food dropped from 42 percent in 1900 to 30 percent in 1950, 13.5 percent in 2003, and by 2019, it had shrunk further to just 9.5 percent (USDA, U.S. Department of Agriculture). This abundance of food in the United States, and in many other industrialized nations provided their populations with an opportunity humans had never previously known: "to eat food merely for pleasure and to consume more than the body needed to survive."[96]

An opportunity many of us were more than happy to seize.

Analysis of national food supply data from the U.S. Department of Agriculture (USDA) reveals that per capita food consumption began to rise in the middle of the last century, particularly accelerating in the past five decades. For example, between 1980 and 2000—when obesity in the US started to spike— the average daily caloric intake per person increased by 20 percent, from 2,200 to just over 2,700 calories. That's an additional 500 calories per person each day—roughly the equivalent of one Big Mac.

And so, while many of us may be reluctant to admit it, the growing body of evidence confirms a simple truth: "We're fat because we eat a lot—a whole lot more than we used to."[97]

How Energy *Output* Changed

The recent rise in the population's caloric intake—not only in the US, but pretty much worldwide—could very well have been stifled had there been a balancing increase in energy expenditure. Unfortunately, the population's increased energy intake has been accompanied by a decline in energy output, further exacerbating our collective energy surplus. It is a trend that most experts expect will continue.[98]

For most of our long existence as physically active hunter-gatherers, our energy input and energy expenditure through physical activity were inextricably linked. In today's modern societies, however, that natural balance has been disturbed.

> The convenient modern world has virtually eliminated the evolutionary connection between energy expenditure and calorie ingestion. The "search and pursuit" time (to hunt, gather, forage, and fish) are minimized, while the caloric payoff is almost unlimited. Today, the acquisition of massive amounts of calorie-dense foods and beverages requires minimal energy expenditure. This systematic and pervasive disconnect between energy intake and energy expenditure inherent in modern cultures is a fundamental factor in the obesity epidemic.[99]

In gradual, often subtle ways, physical exertion continues to be engineered out of our modern lifestyle. Whether on the farm, in the factory, at the office, or at home, technology increasingly performs tasks that our bodies once did.

As advanced economies shift from an emphasis on the production of goods to the provision of services, fewer people are working in jobs that are "sweat-friendly." Recent U.S. census data shows that the proportion of the workforce employed in occupations requiring heavy manual labor—

such as farming, masonry, carpentry, and industrial factory work—continues to decline, while the share working in more sedentary white-collar jobs is rising. Many of these service-oriented jobs, in fields like banking, insurance, health, and education, demand little physical effort, often requiring no more than pressing keys on a computer.[100,101]

Even in traditionally labor-intensive environments like farms and factories, modern labor-saving technologies are increasingly taking over tasks that once relied on human muscle.[102] It is estimated that a century ago, as much as 30 percent of the energy used in farm and factory work came from muscle power; today, that number has dropped to just one percent.[103]

The forces driving these trends are not just technological; they are economic as well. As is often said, "Economics craft institutions into energy-saving enterprises."[104] In many industries, minimizing physical labor and replacing it with technology has proven to be an effective cost-saving strategy. While this has been beneficial for our wallets, it has also had profound and unintended consequences on the economic incentives that drive us to burn calories.

Simply put, when work was physically demanding, we were, in effect, *getting paid to exercise*. Today, as more jobs become increasingly sedentary, we must pay for physical activity[105]—not only in the money we pay to get into the gym, but in foregone leisure time.[106] In today's society, burning significant calories often means choosing between going to the gym or spending time with our spouse or kids.[107]

At home, the growing reliance on prepared foods and the proliferation of labor-saving appliances—such as washing machines, dishwashers, and self-propelled lawn mowers—have led to a significant decline in household-related physical work, further exacerbating the problem.[108]

It is all adding up to an environment where fewer of us are expending the energy necessary to compensate for our growing appetites.[109]

As a result of all of this, energy expenditure for most adults in the U.S. rarely rises above the *resting level*—equivalent to between 60 and 100 watts, the energy output of an ordinary light bulb! No wonder, U.S. citizens have aptly been dubbed *homo sedentarius*.[110]

A Sad Irony

Taken together, the emerging picture reveals a confluence of multiple factors—agriculture, technology, and socioeconomic forces—that are reinforcing each other, transforming our environment from one where work was strenuous and food scarce to one where energy expenditure is low and food is abundant.[111]

It is a sad irony. The very modern environment we worked so hard to create—while undeniably comfortable—is one that our body's Pleistocene-era energy-regulating system was not designed for. And an increasing number of people are paying the price.[112]

In the remainder of this chapter, I explain how *asymmetry* is physiologically wired into the human energy regulation system, not just to regulate energy input, but also for regulating energy expenditure and storage.

Three Asymmetries in Human Energy Regulation

Because ensuring adequate energy for survival and reproduction is crucial, our body does not leave energy metabolism to chance. An energy deficit could mean not only a failure to thrive but, in many cases, a threat to survival.[113] To prevent this, a multitude of overlapping physiological pathways regulate energy input, expenditure, and storage ensuring an adequate supply of long-term energy resources for survival and reproduction.

Asymmetry in Energy-Input (EI) Regulation

When most of us think about our food intake or appetite, we tend to focus on the short-term—meal to meal or day to day. Cultural and social conventions significantly influence not only the food we choose to eat, but also the size, timing, and composition of our meals. As a result, food intake often seems like a behavior that is under voluntary control. While this is partly true, it is far from the whole story. Metabolic and physiologic mechanisms play a major, albeit less visible, role in regulating our energy intake.

Experimental research conducted over the past half-century has shown that the initiation and termination of feeding are complex processes, involving both reflective and reflexive components. Like other forms of human behavior, eating is an activity that is orchestrated and mediated by the brain.[114] Incoming signals from diverse sources within and outside the body are integrated in a small region at the base of the brain called the hypothalamus, where they are processed to ultimately trigger or suppress appetite. (Complementary animal studies have demonstrated that placing tiny lesions in this area can cause obesity or leanness, depending on the location of the lesions.[115])

The emerging model of the *biological* drivers of human food intake (which themselves, as we shall see, are not the sole drivers), suggests that they are controlled by two regulatory subsystems: one short-term and the other long-term. The short-term subsystem aims to provide energy substrates to meet the immediate metabolic needs of the body by controlling the onset and cessation of feeding on a meal-to-meal basis. After a large meal, the unused portion of ingested food energy is stored, primarily in the body's fat reserves. The long-term regulatory component monitors the depletion or repletion of these reserves. The brain plays a critical role in both subsystems.

Recent advances in functional Magnetic Resonance Imaging (fMRI), magnetoencephalography (MEG), and electroencephalography (EEG) have enabled considerable research into the signals that shuttle between the brain, stomach, and fat reserves to regulate these subsystems. Scientists now have a much clearer understanding of how: (1) incoming signals from various sources within the body are integrated in the brain to create a real-time picture of the body's energy status, and (2) how the brain responds by orchestrating output messages to trigger or suppress appetite.[116]

The Short-term Subsystem As mentioned, the short-term component regulates the onset and cessation of feeding on a meal-to-meal basis. During the course of a meal, the body relies on an extensive array of receptors along the gastrointestinal tract to relay information to the brain about the amount and nutrient content of the food, so that the meal may be terminated when sufficient food has been consumed.[117,118]

Here's how this short-term subsystem works: as food enters the gastrointestinal (GI) tract, mechano-receptors in the stomach detect the stretch caused by the food, sending signals to the brain about how much food has been ingested. Simultaneously, the different nutrients in the ingested food interact with chemo-receptors along the small intestine, triggering the release of gastrointestinal hormones such as cholecystokinin, which signal the nutrient content of the meal. These neuronal and hormonal signals are then processed in the brain's feeding-control center within the hypothalamus, tracking both the amount of food eaten and its nutrient content, while orchestrating the feelings of hunger and satiation that drive us to continue or stop eating.[119]

Within the hypothalamus, specifically in the arcuate nucleus (ARC), energy and feeding status indicators from these various sources influence neurons responsible for regulating appetite. Stimulation of these neurons creates feelings of hunger or fullness and ultimately triggers the start or stop of eating. For instance, when the appetite-related neurons are activated by an empty stomach, the ARC releases appetite-stimulating peptides such as neuropeptide Y (NPY), promoting hunger and eating.[120] Conversely, after food consumption, signals from the stomach and intestine activate a different set of neurons, the satiety-related group, producing the opposite, anorexigenic effect— reducing appetite and signaling fullness.[121]

Over the last two decades, pioneering research by Dr. Barbara Rolls and her team at Pennsylvania State University has demonstrated that food volume has "the overriding influence" on satiety.[122] In other words, it's the physical bulk of food, rather than its caloric content, that contributes most to the signals sent to the brain, letting us know we've had enough. In controlled lab experiments, the Rolls team found that participants consistently consumed a fixed volume of food per meal to feel satisfied, regardless of its caloric content.[123] (In our "natural" environment—where we are constantly tempted to snack on this or taste that— people tend to show greater variability in their food intake from meal to meal and day to day. For instance, research indicates that we typically consume more food on days when we eat out.) However, when scientists examine the biological drivers of food intake in controlled lab settings, they consistently find that the total weight of food a person consumes remains remarkably stable from day to day. This suggests that we have learned how much bulk it takes to satisfy our hunger, and that is what we choose to eat.[124]

Why would our system evolve to monitor bulk rather than the energy or nutrient content of food? Researchers Blundell and King from the BioPsychology Group at the University of Leeds offer a compelling theory: historically, before the advent of processed foods, the weight and volume of food were often reliable indicators of its energy value and nutrient content. Over time, our bodies adapted to use weight and volume as subconscious cues for gauging a meal's nutritional worth. This (over)reliance on bulk as a proxy for nutritional value is a logical adaptation that our bodies continue to use today.[125]

The meal's bulk required to reach satiety varies from person to person and even for each individual over time. Rather than being a fixed figure like 800 grams, it falls within a range, as research from Cornell University's Food and Brand Lab has demonstrated.[126] Their studies suggest that most people are content eating meals that lie within what they termed the "satiated margin"—a range that satisfies without prompting noticeable concern over small differences in meal weight. When we eat within this margin, we feel satisfied and remain indifferent to minor variations in portion size.

Human appetite, in other words, is not only asymmetric, it is also elastic. Another functional adaptation that also served us well over the eons of human existence. An elastic appetite would have allowed our hunter gather ancestors to be perfectly *comfortable* overeating whenever the opportunity presented itself, allowing them to build up those reserves of fat that sustained them during periods of food deprivation.[127] (In today's age of abundant and tempting fast food, this elasticity has become a double-edged sword, however, as discussed further in the chapter's appendix on the *reward* of food.)

A feeding episode—a meal—provides the energy needed to meet the body's immediate metabolic demands. After a large meal, the unused portion of ingested food energy is stored, primarily as fat. The function of the second (long-term) regulatory component is to monitor the depletion and repletion of these fat reserves, a crucial function for both survival and efficient functioning.

The Long-Term Subsystem. To stay alive, humans, like all living organisms, need to continuously expend energy—literally every second of every day, whether awake or asleep. This energy fuels not only physical activity but also the body's essential metabolic and internal housekeeping functions such as breathing, heartbeats, blood cell renewal, and waste filtration. Our capacity to store energy long-term, primarily as fat, is what allows us to expend energy *continuously*, without needing to refuel every moment.

Imagine the inconvenience if we lacked this capacity. Without storage, energy output would have to align exactly with energy intake, demanding constant feeding. Thankfully, our ability to store energy decouples energy-in from energy-out, allowing us to eat only a few times daily, with each meal covering immediate needs and creating reserves for later.

Beyond the obvious convenience that this provides us on a day-to-day basis, our capacity to store energy is also key to our survival in a food-scarce environment.[128] Unlike marine species with constant access to nutrients, like oysters that passively filter food from seawater, humans evolved to conserve energy as a buffer against unpredictable food availability.[129] As author Sharman Russell noted, this allowed our ancestor to survive not just a bad day of hunting, but a bad week of hunting and not just a bad crop, but a bad year of crops.[130]

For species without constant access to food, conserving excess energy—primarily in the form of adipose tissue—is a necessary survival characteristic. (Adipose, which is another word for fatty, comes from the Latin *adipatus,* meaning "greasy."[131,132]) Species such as humans... and the polar bear.

> The main energy source of the polar bear is seal meat. The bear can only catch seals during the winter when the animals surface at the breathing openings in the ice. During the summer, with less ice, the polar bear cannot catch the seals, which are much more skillful swimmers than are bears. Throughout the winter the bears accumulate a massive amount of adipose tissue by preferentially selecting to eat the fat-rich parts of the seals such as the brains of

the lean seal pups. The stored fat is then used for survival during the summer.[133]

Like the polar bear, humans evolved to store energy primarily as fat—a choice that was no evolutionary accident. Fat is remarkably efficient, providing more than twice the energy per gram compared to protein or carbohydrate (nine kilocalories per gram of fat versus four per gram of protein or carbohydrate).[134] This high energy density allows for substantial energy reserves with minimal bulk, providing a critical advantage to our ancestors who had to be highly motile to survive.[135]

Even today, this energy efficiency serves us well. For instance, a young woman typically carries enough fat to sustain her for one to two months. If she were to store the same amount of energy as carbohydrate, she would probably be too bulky to walk.[136] Fat's compact energy storage thus remains a vital adaptation, even in the 21st century.

The level of body fat for any individual is the cumulative sum of the differences between energy intake and energy expenditure. To regulate this energy store at desired levels, the brain must perform two vital functions. First, it must sense the size of the fat stores and, second, it must be able to adjust hunger, satiety and energy expenditure as needed.[137] To do that, the brain relies on a lot of help from the body's fat mass.

The body's fat stores are far from the passive receptacles they were once believed to be. Rather, the body's fat cells are highly active tissue that spins out a steady supply of nearly a dozen hormones—collectively known as adipokines—that carry messages to the brain and the rest of the body.[138] Because the concentration of these hormonal signals corresponds to the amount of stored fat, they provide a reliable gauge of the body's energy reserves.

When the brain detects a change in the status of the body's energy reserves—say a drop below desired levels—it triggers compensatory responses to adjust food intake and energy output. An increase or decrease in intake, for example, can be induced by adjusting the frequency and/or size of meals. This is achieved through the release of brain peptides like neuropeptide Y from the hypothalamus that serve to enhance or decrease the potency of the short-term satiety (or meal-ending) signals to the brain. In other words, the size of the fat reserves can turn up or turn down the *sensitivity* of the brain to the meal-generated satiety signals—which, as explained above, are part of the short-term regulatory subsystem. It is an elegant two-tier system, and it works.

> [A]n individual who has recently eaten insufficient food to maintain its weight will be less sensitive to meal-ending signals and, given the opportunity, will consume larger meals on the average. Analogously, an individual who has enjoyed excess food and consequently gained some weight will, over time, become more sensitive to meal-terminating signals.[139]

This system of feeding regulation is inherently asymmetric. When fat stores decrease due to a sustained energy deficit, the neuronal and hormonal signals that stimulate feeding are more potent than the inhibitory signals produced when fat stores increase through overfeeding. This imbalance ensures a stronger drive to eat in response to energy loss than to refrain from eating when energy stores are abundant.

This was demonstrated more than thirty years ago in a clever series of experiments designed to reveal the differences in how humans compensate for increases and decreases in the energy content of their diet. In the experiments, Mattes et al.[140] surreptitiously diluted and then boosted the energy content of meals offered to free-living experimental subjects and observed how they compensated. What they found was rather surprising. When their subjects received lunches containing 66 percent fewer calories than their customary midday meal, the subjects compensated for the lunch-time deficit by ingesting additional non-lunch calories. As a result, their total energy intakes did not decrease. In contrast, when the subjects were covertly provided lunches containing 66 percent more calories than their customary midday meal, they did not adjust their non-lunch energy intake downward to compensate. As a result, total energy intake was significantly higher.

Humans appear to be biologically "wired" to aggressively compensate for caloric deprivation, but not for minor caloric surpluses. Our understanding of the biological underpinnings of this asymmetry in our regulatory system was significantly advanced by the discovery of leptin in 1994. Leptin is an amino acid protein synthesized in fat cells and secreted into the blood stream in concentrations that are proportional to total fat stores. As such, it serves as a primary signaling mechanism to the brain about how much fat the body has stored.

Research has shown that "when a person's fat stores shrink, so does (the body's) leptin production. In response, appetite increases while metabolism decreases."[141] The system, however, does not work quite the same in the other direction; that is, a rise in leptin does not necessarily lead to appetite reduction.[142] The experimental evidence "exposes" the brain's true intentions in deploying leptin: it deploys it to track how much fat the body has stored *not to keep us from getting fat, but to keep us from getting too thin.*[143]

In summary, several principles may be deduced about human appetite regulation: 1) Feeding is controlled by two regulatory subsystems, one short- and the other long-term; 2) The two systems are physiologically interdependent; and 3) the two-tier system is asymmetric.

Asymmetry in Energy-Expenditure (EE) Regulation

To adequately manage the body's energy reserves, it is not enough that the regulatory system manages the amount of energy input into the body. Just as in managing the financial budget of a business or a household, one needs to keep an eye on both sides of the ledger—what is coming in and what is going out. And so, with human energy regulation, the system needs to also oversee how energy is consumed and stored. This section discusses energy consumption, and the next explains how the body manages the status of its energy stores.

Total energy expenditure is generally divided into three components. The smallest, comprising about 10 percent, is the energy used to process the food we eat—its digestion and absorption. A second component is the energy expended for muscular work. This typically accounts for 15 to 20 percent of daily energy expenditure, but can increase by a factor of two or more with heavy physical exertion.[144] The third and largest component is basal energy expenditure—also known as maintenance (or resting) energy expenditure (MEE)—which is the energy required to keep us alive. This is the amount of energy required for the basic maintenance of the cells and sustaining the essential physiological functions—to pump blood, regulate temperature, breathe, or think. For most of us, the MEE makes up about 60 to 70 percent of total energy expenditure.

The body's regulatory system for energy expenditure evolved to complement the over-consumption bias (as explained above). It achieves this by reducing metabolic rate in response to a negative energy balance and by favoring energy conservation when physical activity isn't required.[145] As Polivy and Herman argue, it is an effective strategy for ensuring the body's fuel reserves are preserved during lean times:

> If there is a dearth of food available, the organism is better served by physiological adjustments that render what *is* available more useful—by means of what has come to be known as a *thrifty* metabolism—rather than by promptings to acquire more food when there simply is no more to be acquired, or when the energy expended in acquiring more might well exceed the energy content of the food itself. In short, in an ecology of scarcity, we are better served by metabolic adjustments than by behavioral adjustments.[146]

As soon as the body senses an energy deficit, basal metabolism drops quite dramatically in order to conserve energy and restrain the rate of tissue loss. This is achieved chiefly through hormonal mechanisms that operate to decrease the metabolic activity at the cellular level, in essence enhancing the tissues' metabolic efficiency—much like switching to energy-saving fluorescent light bulbs to reduce power consumption.[147] (For example, muscle biopsies taken before, during and after weight loss show that once a person drops weight, their muscle fibers undergo a transformation, making them more like highly efficient "slow twitch" muscle fibers that burn 20 to 25 percent fewer calories during everyday activity.[148]) This homeostatic mechanism serves as a first line of defense against energy imbalance—a buffer, if you will, that helps spare the body's fat reserves in lean times. While this may be frustrating for dieters today (because it limits weight loss), the survival value of an energy-sparing regulatory process that aims to limit tissue depletion during food scarcity is clear.

The body's regulatory mechanisms work in reverse when confronted with a positive energy balance. Sort of. When sustained positive energy balance leads to weight gain, the body's maintenance energy expenditure (MEE) does increase—but only modestly. Experimental studies of human energy regulation reveal that, in this less threatening scenario, the body's biological signals remain relatively "muted."[149] Although MEE adjusts upward when in positive energy balance, the adjustments do not increase energy expenditures enough to fully compensate for the imbalance.

The system clearly is not as robustly organized to galvanize in response to energy surpluses (which pose minimal survival threat) as it is for deficits (which pose a significant threat). This asymmetry in energy expenditure aligns with the intake-side bias we observed earlier. Working in concert, these two limbs of our body's energy regulation system have effectively evolved us into what we are today: "exquisitely efficient calorie conservation machines."[150]

Asymmetry in Energy-Storage Regulation

In addition to the asymmetry in regulating energy intake and expenditure, there is a third form of asymmetry related to energy storage: the system has a built-in bias to tolerate—and favor—the build-up of energy reserves... but not their depletion.

The food we eat—our primary energy source—provides three energy-yielding macronutrients: protein, carbohydrate, and fat. Proteins primarily serve as the building blocks for body tissue,[151] while fats and carbohydrates act as the body's main fuels, powering biological functions and physical activity.

When food is ingested, the chemical energy trapped within the bonds of the food nutrients is initially stored in the body's tissues. This stored energy is then converted by the musculoskeletal system into mechanical energy, with some of it inevitably transformed into heat, or used for building body structures. If we consume more calories than we expend, or are insufficiently active, the excess energy is stored in the body's reserves.

By a large margin, the primary form in which the body stores excess energy from food is fat, stored in specialized fat cells called adipocytes. This conferred evolutionary advantages since, as was mentioned, fat is the more efficient way to store energy, storing nearly two and a half times as many calories per gram as glycogen—the storage form of carbohydrates. "In lean adults, fat reserves typically amount to some 10 kg, an energy reserve of 90,000 kcal, enough to survive about two months of near total food deprivation."[152] By contrast, the average person has only about 2,500 calories stored as carbohydrates, primarily in the liver and muscle.

The human body's capacity to store excess calories as fat is truly remarkable.[153] Over a lifetime, an extremely obese person might accumulate 300 to 400 pounds of fat, enough to fuel the body's energy needs for a year or more. ("Medical journals tell of one 450-pound man who fasted under medical supervision for a year and two weeks, taking nothing but zero-calorie liquids, and lost nearly 280 pounds without any ill effects."[154])

The total amount of fat in a person's body is a function of and is regulated by two factors: the number of fat cells and their size. During periods of positive energy balance and weight gain, excess energy is initially stored in the body's existing fat cells, causing them to expand. While fat cells can enlarge considerably, they have a biological limit of about 1.0 microgram (μg) of fat.[155] Once they reach this peak size, a process of fat cell proliferation is initiated, ultimately increasing the body's total fat cell number.[156] Obesity, thus, develops when a person's fat cells increase in number, in size, or, quite often, both. Importantly, once fat cells are created, their number seems to remain fixed, even if weight is lost.[157,158] That is, with weight loss, cells shrink, but do not decrease in number.[159,160,161]

This was demonstrated in a study that tracked the change in adipose tissue profiles of 19 obese adults as they reduced their body mass from an average of 149 kg (328 lb.) to 103 kg (227 lb.) during a weight-loss program (Figure 3.3). The average number of fat cells remained steady at 75 billion, even after a 46-kg (101 lb.) reduction in body weight. However, fat cell size decreased from 0.9 to 0.6 micrograms (μg) of lipid per cell—a reduction of 33 percent. The authors concluded that, "a shrinkage of adipocytes with no change in cell number is the major change in adipose cellularity following weight loss in adults."[162,163]

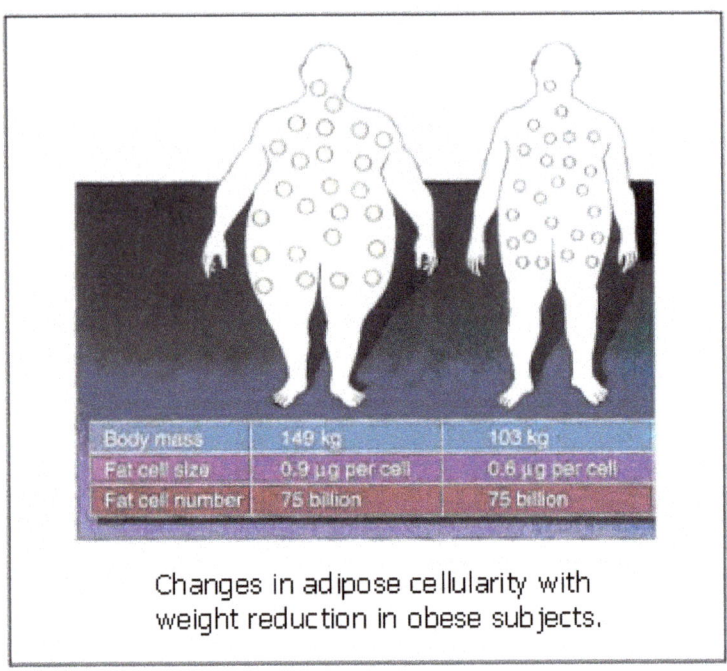

Figure 3.3
Adipose cellularity

The lifecycle of fat cells paints a discouraging picture for those who are significantly overweight. With each increase in body weight, new fat cells may form—and once created, they are nearly impossible to eliminate.[164] Furthermore, according to fat-cell theory (discussed below), the body strives to maintain a normal fat-cell size. As a result, the increased number of fat cells that often accompanies significant weight gain not only raises body weight but also prompts the body to defend that weight. This biological trap has profound implications for energy balance and weight regulation. Let's take a closer look.

"Biological Trap" for Dieters. The way the body regulates its energy stores differs in a very significant way from other *homeostatic processes* that maintain stable levels of various physiological variables despite environmental changes. (Homeostasis—self-regulation—is a fundamental property of all self-organizing systems to preserve balance in response to environmental shifts.) For example, consider core body temperature: the system's <u>target</u> remains constant at 98.6°F, regardless of ambient temperature or activity level. If body temperature begins to rise say during exercise or drop after a plunge into cold water, the body initiates corrective actions, like sweating or shivering, to bring core temperature back to the desired level.

In the case of regulating fat storage, by contrast, the system's target is *not* static (as with desired body temperature). Instead, the set point that regulates the size of the energy reserves is a *moving target* that can ratchet up over time. In this case, a <u>dynamic</u> control scheme was obviously necessary to allow for the natural growth in body weight from childhood through adulthood. (The number of fat cells increases gradually and continuously through childhood and adolescence as the body naturally grows in size, increasing in number approximately fivefold between the ages of one and twenty for a non-obese individual.[165,166]) In addition, such an adaptive control scheme would have conferred a survival advantage throughout human prehistory, allowing for the buildup of energy reserves in times of plenty.

A key regulator in setting and resetting this moving target is fat-cell size.[167] According to fat-cell theory, the body strives to maintain *normal* fat cell size.[168] Research in fat-tissue cellularity is beginning to clarify how fat cells communicate their size status to the brain. This mechanism resembles how mechano-receptors in the gastrointestinal tract detect stomach distension and relay information about nutrient levels to the brain. As fat cells expand with stored fat, the stretching of their membranes—and the resulting increase in membrane tension—signals the brain about their size. Both hormonal and enzymatic mechanisms on the fat cell membranes appear to play roles in this signaling process.[169,170]

To illustrate how the various components of this regulatory scheme interact—how weight gain influences fat cell number and size, which, in turn, adjusts the body's set point—let's examine a hypothetical example. Consider the case of an average male, "Mr. Average," or "Mr. A" for short. He is six feet tall and weighs 180 pounds, which gives him a body mass index (BMI) of 24—calculated by dividing weight in kilograms by the square of height in meters. A fat-tissue analysis reveals that his body contains 25 billion fat cells, each averaging 0.5 µg in size.

Mr. A's weight has remained relatively steady over the last few years. Like most of us, he has experienced occasional, modest fluctuations, sometimes gaining, sometimes losing a few pounds, but always managing to revert back to what he considers his "normal" weight. However, a change in lifestyle—perhaps a move to the city, a job change, or a shift in family dynamics—leads him into an extended period of positive energy balance (e.g., sustained nutritional excess and/or reduced physical activity). A year later, when we revisit him, we find that he has gained 40 pounds.

To accommodate his increased fat mass, Mr. A's fat cells would have expanded in size and increased in number. However, this process does not occur uniformly throughout the body, as newly stored fat is never distributed evenly among the body's fat stores. Fat deposition is modulated by enzymes, such as the enzyme lipoprotein lipase (LPL), found on the membranes of fat cell. The activity of LPL is partially controlled by sex-specific hormones—estrogen in women and testosterone in men. In men, for example, fat cells in the abdomen produce an abundance of LPL, and, as a result, men tend to store fat there and develop central obesity.[171]

Unhappy with his expanding waistline, Mr. A decides to go on a diet to lose weight—and he succeeds. His goal is to return to 180 pounds, the weight he once considered "normal" before his recent (and, he hopes, temporary) weight gain. Unfortunately for Mr. A, the weight gain and the accompanying changes at the cellular level in his body are not entirely transient or reversible. As some of his fat cells grew and divided—particularly in areas where fat accumulation was more pronounced—his fat cell count would have increased, say, to 28 billion. As a result, when he starts losing the weight, the "I am at target level" signal from the body's energy stores to the brain will now correspond to a higher weight—one associated with 28 billion cells, each averaging 0.5 µg. This will occur when his body weight is around 200 pounds. Dropping below this newly elevated *target* weight—say, back to his original 180 pounds—will cause these 28 billion fat cells to shrink to a size smaller than 0.5 µg. The body will interpret this shrinkage as a depletion of energy reserves below "desired" level, triggering hormonal signals to the brain to scream, "Eat, eat, eat!"[172]

The bottom line is this: gaining a <u>significant</u> amount of weight leads to irreversible anatomical and physiological changes that cause the body's energy reserves to be regulated at a higher set point. Specifically, fat cell theory posits that the body's *dynamic* set point for energy regulation is determined by the size of fat cells, with the weight at which this occurs depending on their number. Weight loss beyond the point where fat cells return to their normal size would signal a depletion of energy reserves below "desired," inducing overeating to refill the fat cells.[173,174]

Thus, fat-cell size and number together modulate eating so as to maintain total fat stores while striving to keep fat-cell size at some normal level. This dynamic mechanism sets and resets the body's energy regulation set point. Since the body strives to achieve and maintain normal fat-cell size, the increased number of fat cells that typically accompanies excessive weight gain not only elevates body weight but also defends that weight. In this way, appetite doesn't just shape body weight; growing body weight also influences appetite!

The significance of this for weight maintenance and obesity prevention is clear: It is crucial to intervene before <u>excessive</u> weight is gained and fat-cell proliferation sets in. Otherwise, we risk falling into a "biological trap:" becoming fat from eating too much and continuing to eat too much because our bodies seek to maintain the higher weight associated with the elevated number of fat cells.

Appendix

Beyond Physiology: The *Reward* of Food

In this Chapter, I focused on the *biological drivers* of feeding regulation. While physiological states of need play a leading role, it is far from a solo-act. Over the past half-century, an abundance of research has shown that the initiation and cessation of eating is a complex bio-psychological process, part reflexive and part reflective. Signals from various sources, both within and outside the body, are integrated in the brain to trigger or suppress appetite, driving us to start or stop eating.

We might like to think that we eat only when we're hungry and stop when we're full, but it doesn't work that way. Everyday experience reveals a seemingly trivial fact that, "... people often eat more of better-liked foods when offered an ad libitum choice, and that the experience or anticipation of highly liked food can stimulate its consumption *in the absence of an energy deficit or perceived state of hunger* (italics added)."[175] Overeating when palatable foods are abundant is not unique to humans. Most mammals will eat beyond their needs when presented with foods that are highly appetizing.[176] For example, when wild primates—the mammalian taxon humans belong to—are placed in environments where palatable food is always abundant overeat their way to obesity. (In one study, female baboons in such an environment had 50% greater body mass and 23% body fat, compared with just 2% body fat in their wild-feeding counterparts.[177])

What drives humans and other animals to ignore satiety signals and eat more than they need—or more than is optimal?

In one word: *reward*.

The *Reward* of Food

Five decades into the obesity epidemic, the powerful influence of reward on feeding behavior can no longer be argued.[178] In our modern food-abundant environment, food consumption—not to mention *over*consumption—is rarely induced by acute energy deprivation.[179] The evidence—substantial and growing—indicates that in well-nourished populations, the primary stimulus for eating is increasingly the gratification derived from food, rather than energy deficit.

The human energy regulation system, it is becoming increasingly clear, does not function as a purely physiological process. Rather, it is a complex biopsychological phenomenon, shaped by interactions between physiological homeostatic processes and the reward (or hedonic) effects of food. This is not to say that food deprivation is not a powerful motivator of eating—both in humans and animals. It is. And it likely always will be. However, in our modern environment of abundance, the hunger-induced physiological drive to seek food is becoming increasingly secondary.

According to the emerging positive-incentive theory, people in modern industrialized societies are not primarily motivated to eat by the decline of their energy reserves below set points. Rather, they are drawn to eat by the anticipated pleasure of eating—the positive-incentive value of food.

> People will consume highly palatable foods when such foods are available because they have evolved to find pleasure in this behavior. Positive-incentive theorists do not deny that major reductions in the body's energy resources below homeostatic levels increase hunger, as well as eating, if food is available. They do, however, view this relation differently than do set-point theorists. According to set-point theory, reduction of the body's energy resources below energy set points is the main motivating factor in food consumption; according to positive-incentive theory, humans and other animals living in food-replete environments rarely, if ever, experience an energy deficit. This is because they find the consumption of high positive-incentive value foods so rewarding that when such foods are readily available, they consume far more than they need to meet their energy requirements.[180]

Humans—and animals—will work for food, illustrating how rewards motivate behavior: they engage in activities not directly related to food and stop once they receive the reward. In fact, many of us willingly spend large sums for an exceptional meal, and nearly any mammal will consume beyond its homeostatic needs when offered highly palatable food.[181]

Many factors interact to influence the positive incentive value of food, with individual differences at play. For most people, however, the anticipated <u>taste</u> of food stands out as one of the most significant factors:

> [People develop] a relish for particular tastes that are in nature associated with foods that promote human survival. For example, humans normally develop a liking for sweet, fatty, and salty tastes—tastes that in nature are usually characteristic of foods that are rich in energy and essential vitamins and minerals... Superimposed on these species-characteristic taste preferences and aversions are individual preferences and aversions that each person develops through interactions with other members of the species and through experiencing the health-promoting and health-disrupting effects of the foods he or she eats.[182]

But does reward-driven eating <u>override</u> the drive for satiety and promote overeating? The evidence suggests the answer is yes—the drive for reward can indeed dominate the drive for satiation and balance. Sometimes aggressively so.[183] In a recent study, for example, "81% of respondents reported that in situations in which they have access to a large supply of preferred foods, they frequently (overeat) until they feel ill."[184]

In major new research thrust, scientists are seeking to understand how the liking and wanting of food work together to affect the reinforcing value of food and ultimately contribute to overeating behavior. Central to this research is neuroscience, which is shedding light on the brain's neurotransmitter systems that orchestrate the workings of this feeding-related reward system.

Research has shown that food rewards and drug rewards share common neural pathways, with opioid receptors playing a central role in both systems. It seems no coincidence that the term "craving" describes intense desires for both palatable foods and addictive substances.[185] Studies comparing sugar-rich diets to those with artificial sweeteners have demonstrated that it is the palatability of food—not its energy content—that activates the brain's opioid system.[186] Furthermore, evidence suggests that the brain's endogenous opioid systems regulate the hedonic value of food intake independently of the body's metabolic needs.[187] This suggests that, due to the high priority of feeding, mammalian brains have developed multiple overlapping neuronal systems that potentiate eating behavior.[188]

A hallmark of behavior driven by the brain's reward circuitry—mediated by endogenous opioids, dopamine, and serotonin—is the persistent desire to "come back for more."

> Whether the opioid circuits are activated by highly palatable foods or by drugs, they enable the body to perceive a rewarding experience... A highly palatable food tells the brain, 'This is a desirable object, get more'...
> [Case in point:] Martin Yeomans at the University of Sussex, in England, has done experiments in which he keeps interrupting people as they eat to ask them how hungry they are. Halfway through their meals some people rate their hunger levels higher than before they started to eat.[189]

Another explanation for overeating palatable foods comes from animal studies, which show that diets high in fat and sugar can blunt the brain's satiety signals. In experiments with mice, it was found that satiety hormones such as cholecystokinin and leptin were suppressed on these high-fat, high-sugar diets. This suppression led to longer meals and, ultimately, overeating and increased fat accumulation.[190] See sidebar.

> A new study suggests that (Oreos)"America's favorite cookie" is just as addictive as cocaine or morphine -- at least in lab rats.
> Researchers found that in lab rats, eating Oreos activated more neurons in the brain's "pleasure center" than exposure to drugs like cocaine and morphine. / Bob MacDonnell, courtesy of Connecticut College.
> A new study suggests that high-fat/high-sugar foods stimulate the brain in the same way that drugs do.
> Researchers also looked in the nucleus accumbens, or the brain's pleasure center, and measured how much c-Fos, a protein marker that signals brain neuron activation, was expressed. In simple terms, they were looking at how many cells were turned on in response to the drugs or Oreos.
> The researchers saw that Oreos activated significantly more neurons than cocaine or morphine.
> This correlated well with previous studies. Previous studies have shown that highly-processed carbohydrates like cakes, cookies and chips could affect this same pleasure center in the brain by triggering the release of dopamine, a neurotransmitter that is released when the brain senses something that is a reward.
> This could explain why people have a hard time turning junk food down. It may explain why some people can't resist these foods despite the fact that they know they are bad for them.
> Overall, it lent support to the hypothesis that high-fat/high-sugar foods can be viewed in the same way as drugs of abuse and have addictive potential.

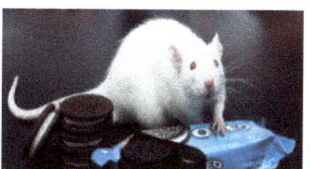

In summary, the following conclusions can be drawn about human appetite regulation: The reward of food is a powerful modulator of feeding behavior, and in an environment abundant with palatable foods, it drives us to eat beyond our needs. As Pine et al. argue, this makes perfect evolutionary sense:

> From the perspective of our evolutionary analysis, the reason humans living in modern industrialized societies tend to overeat is that the presence, the expectation, or even the thought of food with a high positive-incentive value promotes hunger. Because in nature high positive-incentive value foods are rich sources of vitamins, minerals, and energy, it is important that such foods be consumed each time the opportunity presents itself so that the nutrients they provide can be banked as protection against potential future food scarcity.[191]

Part II

Judo-Inspired Weight-Loss Game Plan

Contrary to popular culture—and the widespread yearning for simple, one-size-fits-all solutions—such approaches rarely (if ever) succeed in solving complex challenge. Whether at the individual, organizational, or societal level, simplistic solutions inevitably fall short. This is painfully true for weight loss, which remains an enduring and formidable challenge despite the quick fixes so often touted in the media.

Judo, the antithesis of a "one-trick pony," is a discipline rooted in mastering a broad range of *physical* techniques and cultivating the *mental* agility to adapt and respond. A judoka doesn't rely on brute force when confronting a larger opponent but instead leverages their opponent's energy and movements to gain the upper hand. This adaptability is crucial and, as emphasized in Chapter 2, begins with a deep understanding of the challenge—recognizing your opponent's posture, strengths, and vulnerabilities, and using them to shift the balance. This concept inspired the writing of Chapter 3, where we sought to deepen our understanding of the body's innate energy and weight regulation system—its mechanisms for building energy reserves and defending against depletion.

In keeping with the Judo playbook, our task in Part II is to build a toolkit of Judo-inspired techniques that allow us to manage weight by working with, not against, the body's natural energy-regulation processes. Our goal is ambitious: to develop strategies that not only enable us to manage body weight *efficiently,* but also align with personal lifestyle choices and preferences. These strategies aren't just about losing weight—they are about cultivating sustainable habits that support both weight loss and the <u>prevention</u> of weight gain in an obesogenic environment.

In Judo, techniques are categorized into three main groups, called *waza*: 1) throwing techniques (*nage-waza*), 2) grappling techniques (*katame-waza*), and 3) striking techniques (*atemi-waza*). In Chapters 4 through 7, I will present analogous categories of Judo-inspired *weight-regulation* strategies. These strategies tackle: 1) Managing energy intake by controlling *what* we eat and drink; 2) Managing energy intake by changing *how* we eat; 3) Managing energy expenditure, i.e., how we burn what we consume; and 4) Strategies for deploying our limited self-regulatory energy to stay the course and successfully implement all of the above.

Chapter 4

Managing Energy-In
Part A: *What* we Eat and Drink

Start by Understanding *Satiety*... What Makes Us Feel Full

> *Hunger is the death knell of a weight-loss program.*
> Eric Westman,
> Director, Duke Lifestyle Medicine Clinic

As we explored in Chapter 3, hunger and fullness are governed by two regulatory subsystems—one short-term and the other long-term. The long-term subsystem monitors and regulates the depletion and replenishment of the body's energy reserves. Our focus here is on the short-term component, which regulates *satiation*—the feeling of fullness or nutritional satisfaction during a meal—and signals when eating should stop.

From personal experience we know that,

> [A] full belly is a simple but sure sign that the body has recently taken in energy as food, and [is often the trigger] to reduce appetite. One way that this physical state is communicated to the brain is via distension-sensitive nerve fibers that carry signals from the stomach and intestine, ultimately reaching appetite-control centers.[192]

Perhaps the most enlightening research on the biological regulation of satiation and food intake comes from Dr. Barbara Rolls and her team at Pennsylvania State University. Their pioneering studies, briefly referenced in Chapter 3, demonstrated that food volume—rather than caloric content—is the primary influence on satiety. In other words, it's the bulk of the food, <u>not</u> its caloric content, that signals to our bodies that we've eaten enough.

This finding underscores an important distinction between what makes us feel full—food *bulk*—and what causes us to gain weight—the *energy* content of food. It's a consequential, and potentially empowering, insight. I say "potentially," because it presents dieters with a double-edged sword. Handle the bulk-energy balance wisely, and it's possible to enjoy satisfying meals without gaining weight (if the energy content of those meals is low). But mishandle it, and you may gain weight despite eating smaller, less fulfilling meals (if those meals are energy-dense).

We will opt for wising up!

In this chapter, we'll fully leverage Dr. Rolls's crucial insight into the bulk-energy distinction—not merely to create fulfilling diets for weight loss, but to take it a step further and "cook up" satisfying meals you can genuinely enjoy while shedding pounds. While this may seem like culinary alchemy right now, by the end of the chapter, you'll see how it's entirely feasible to concoct more generous and satisfying meals than the "puny" servings most dieters resign themselves to. All without compromising weight-loss efforts.

The key lies in managing energy density.

The Physics of Energy and Weight *Balance* ain't Complicated

From a physiologic point of view, the basis of weight-gain is no mystery: it arises from a positive *energy* balance. Like all systems—whether technological or biological—the human body adheres to the laws of thermodynamics, which define the immutable principle of energy conservation. Simply put, stored energy—and hence body weight—increases when energy intake exceeds energy expenditure, and decreases when the reverse is true.

Energy in the human body is not self-generated and does not dissipate into biologic black holes; it simply transforms from one form to another. Our primary source of energy is the food we eat—specifically, the chemical energy trapped within the bonds of the food's nutrients such as the proteins, carbohydrates and fats. This ingested energy is then used to accomplish two primary functions: fueling physical activity and sustaining basic metabolic and internal housekeeping processes—such as the synthesis of body tissue, keeping the heart beating, our lungs breathing, and our nerves transmitting.[193] Proteins in the diet primarily provide the building blocks for tissue synthesis, while carbohydrates and fats serve as the body's primary energy sources, fueling both biological functions and physical activity.[194]

If we consume more calories than we expend or are too inactive relative to our intake, the surplus energy is stored in the body's reserves, primarily as fat. This storage of excess energy inevitably leads to weight gain.

Which, if moderate *and* short-term, is not inherently harmful. In fact, our capacity to store energy is what enables us to continuously expend energy—literally every moment of the day—without needing a constant infusion of food. It is also key to our survival when food is scarce. However, when positive energy balance becomes excessive or persistent, it leads to obesity. This is increasingly the case in modern environments, where food is abundant, and physical activity opportunities are shrinking.[195]

As explained in Chapter 3, the body stores excess energy very efficiently—as fat within fat cells, or adipocytes. (Fat is an efficient energy reserve because it contains more than twice the energy per unit weight compared to protein or carbohydrates.) However, no matter how efficiently this storage is accomplished, storing excess energy inevitably leads to increased body weight. For most people, the expansion of fat stores and the resulting weight gain occur gradually over time, typically due to a sustained but modest positive energy balance. This slow upward drift—often just a few pounds per year—is so subtle that it's frequently overlooked or dismissed, even as it steadily contributes to significant weight gain over the years.

A Supposition That Seems Obvious, But Isn't

Most people assume that food energy (calories) increases *automatically and in direct proportion* to amount (or bulk) of food we consume. It seems like an obvious assumption, right?

Wrong.

The reason lies in the fact that different types of food vary significantly in the number of calories they pack into a given weight or volume. In nutritional parlance, this is referred to as energy density (ED), and is defined as the number of calories per gram of food (kcal/g).

$$\text{Energy Density of food} = \frac{Number\ of\ calories}{Weight\ in\ grams}$$

The impact of ED on our diet is best illustrated visually. Consider the two meals shown in Figure 4.1. Both contain 450 calories, but their differences in volume are striking. The top meal—a half cheeseburger, a few fries, and a soda—is markedly smaller in bulk. Because this meal packs the same 450 calories into a smaller volume, its ED is significantly higher than that of the lower meal: an open-faced roast beef sandwich, tomato soup, four-fruit compote, and sparkling water.

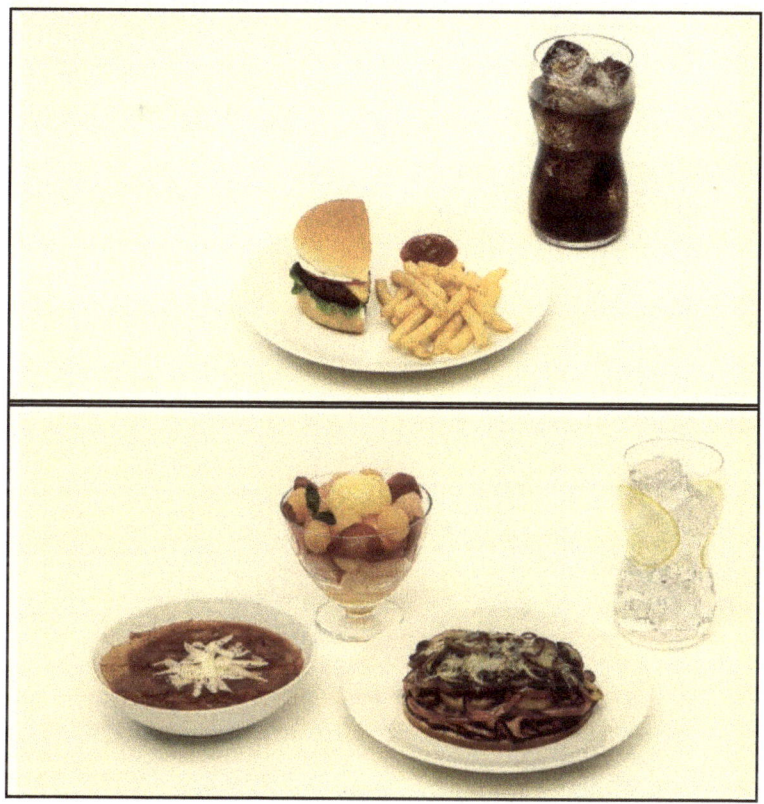

Figure 4.1 Two 450-calorie meals

The smaller, calorie-dense lunch in Figure 4.1 typifies the default calorie-cutting strategy of most dieters: simply eating less of their usual pre-diet meals. In this case, cutting a dieter's usual (pre-diet) burger sandwich by half to reduce calories, say, from 700 to 450. But let's be honest—even in picture form, that half-serving looks unsatisfying, leaving most of us craving more. It's a recipe for frustration and eventual failure.

The mistake? Failing to wisely leverage ED.

If we hope to avoid this all-too-common pitfall, it's crucial to understand the determinants of energy density (ED).

Energy density values are influenced by the macronutrient composition and moisture content of the foods and beverages we consume, with values ranging from 0 kcal/g to 9 kcal/g. That's not a typo—you read that right! There is, indeed, something we consume frequently that has zero calories: water. Since water increases food volume without adding calories, foods with high water content, like vegetables and fruits, allow us to feel full with fewer calories.

This is most clearly illustrated when we compare two similar snacks: grapes and raisins. Both are healthy choices and are essentially the same food—raisins are dried grapes. Figure 4.2 shows what a 100-calorie serving of raisins looks like versus a 100-calorie serving of grapes. If you opt for raisins, you'll only get about ¼ cup, which may leave you still hungry and wanting more. On the other hand, 100 calories of grapes—shown here as about 2 cups—will provide a far more satisfying snack, thanks to their high-water content.

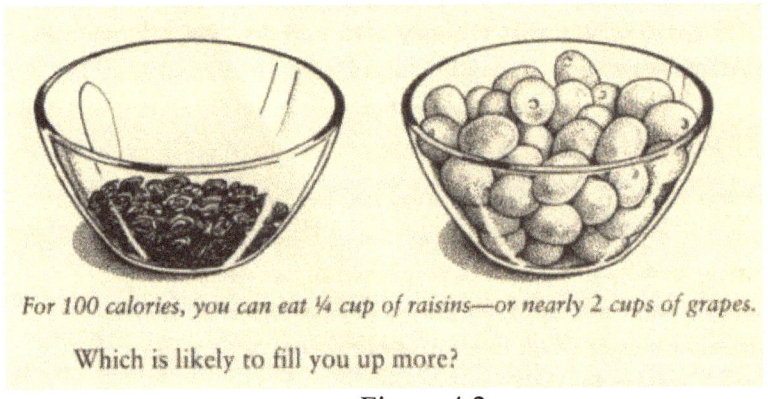

For 100 calories, you can eat ¼ cup of raisins—or nearly 2 cups of grapes.
Which is likely to fill you up more?

Figure 4.2

After water, fiber contributes the most to food volume for the fewest calories—about 1.5 to 2.5 calories per gram. Beyond its impact on energy density (ED), fiber, it's good to know, also offers additional health benefits. See the sidebar for more details.

> ### Fiber's Many Virtues
>
> For years, scientists believed that when it comes to weight gain, all calories are created equal. But a fascinating study by K.D. Corbin et al., published in 2023 in the journal *Nature Communications*, challenges this assumption. The research suggests that the body responds differently to calories from high-fiber whole foods compared to ultra-processed junk foods.
>
> Why? Cheap processed foods are absorbed more quickly in the upper gastrointestinal tract, meaning more calories are available for the body and fewer for the gut microbiome, which resides toward the end of the digestive tract. In contrast, high-fiber foods are less easily absorbed, allowing them to travel the full length of the digestive tract to the large intestine, where trillions of gut bacteria await. By consuming a fiber-rich diet, you're not only nourishing yourself but also your gut microbes, which, according to the new research, effectively reduces your calorie intake.
>
> Our gut microbes thrive on the fibers we eat, breaking them down through fermentation. This process generates beneficial byproducts, such as short-chain fatty acids, which support metabolic health.
>
> The study details an experiment designed to assess the effects of two calorically equivalent diets—one low in fiber, rich in highly processed foods, and the other a high-fiber diet which contained nuts, fruits and vegetables.
>
> The scientists found that the participants absorbed significantly fewer calories on the fiber-rich diet compared to the processed one. Because it requires energy to grow gut bacteria, a portion of ingested energy was expended to expand and nurture the bacteria community instead of going into the participants' energy stores. On average, participants lost 217 calories a day on the fiber-rich diet—about 116 more calories than they lost on the processed-food diet. Furthermore, participants on the fiber-rich diet had higher circulating levels of short-chain fatty acids and increased levels of hormones such as GLP-1, which promotes satiety.
>
> The bottom line: Participants lost slightly more weight and body fat on the fiber-rich diet. Despite absorbing fewer daily calories, they didn't experience increased hunger. This is a remarkable finding because it suggests that people could lose weight and body fat simply by switching to a diet that supports their gut microbiomes—without having to cut back on calories.
>
> Source: The Washington Post, June 13, 2023, *Are all calories created equal? Your gut microbes don't think so*, by Anahad O'Conner.

At the other end of the energy spectrum, dietary fat is the most energy-dense macronutrient, providing more than twice the energy per unit weight compared to protein or carbohydrate (just a quick reminder: 9 calories per gram for fat versus 4 calories per gram for both proteins and carbohydrates). In the "battle of the bulge," fatty foods transform a dinner table into a caloric minefield! Figure 4.3 offers an illustration many of us can relate to: the habitual, almost automatic spreading of butter—a high-fat, energy-dense food we're hardwired to crave—on a slice of bread. As depicted in Figure 4.3, a slice of French bread with 2 teaspoons of butter (with an energy density of 4.0 kcal/g) contains the same number of calories (140 calories) as two slices of bread without butter (ED: 2.75 kcal/g).

High-fat, energy-density foods contribute to weight gain in two primary ways: 1) their higher energy density encourages *passive* overconsumption; and 2) the low thermic effect of fat allows the body to retain more of it.

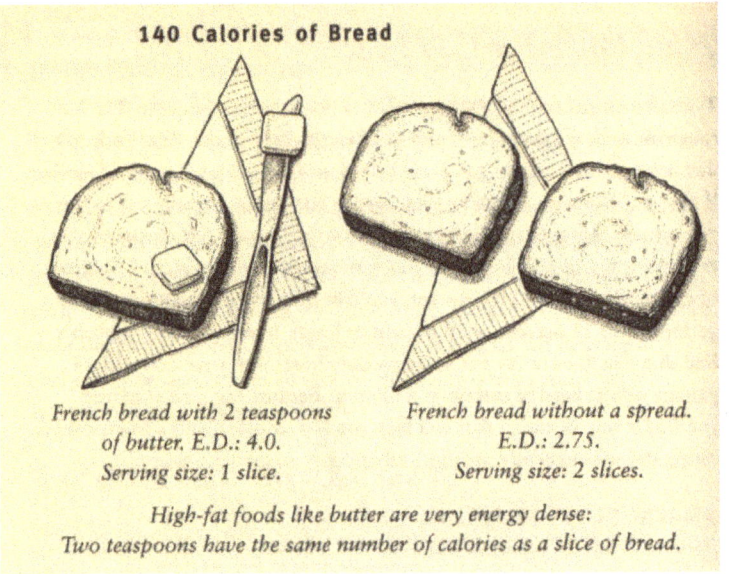

French bread with 2 teaspoons of butter. E.D.: 4.0. Serving size: 1 slice.   *French bread without a spread. E.D.: 2.75. Serving size: 2 slices.*

High-fat foods like butter are very energy dense: Two teaspoons have the same number of calories as a slice of bread.

Figure 4.3

Here's how the first mechanism works: Since—as demonstrated by Dr. Rolls' studies—food volume has "the overriding influence" on satiety, people tend to consume a more or less constant volume of food during a meal to feel full, regardless of its energy content.[196] The corollary, of course, is that when people eat a more or less constant volume of food—the volume that satisfies them—they inadvertently consume more energy (both at a iven meal and throughout the day) when their diets are high in energy density. Because this occurs without conscious effort, the phenomenon has been referred to as *passive* over-consumption.

The second mechanism involves the low thermic effect of fat. What does that mean? When we overeat, the body expends energy to store those extra calories—whether they come from fat, carbohydrates, or proteins—as body fat. The amount of energy expended by the body to digest, absorb, and metabolize the food we eat is referred to as *the thermic effect of food* (TEF). Of the three major macronutrients, fat is stored most efficiently, requiring the least amount of energy to process. This is because the metabolic pathway from dietary fat to body fat involves fewer steps than those for carbohydrates or proteins. For instance, converting excess carbohydrates or proteins into body fat requires about 25 percent of the ingested energy. In contrast, fat is converted with less than 5 percent of the energy being expended.[197] So, when we consume excess calories from fat-rich foods, our bodies tend to retain more of the calories.

The *Judo-esque* Weight-Loss Move

To a *Judoka*, the implication is clear: If people are content with consuming a consistent volume of food at each meal, then less total energy would be automatically (and effortlessly) consumed when one's diet is designed to be low in energy density. This can be achieved, for example, by replacing energy-dense foods like butter, full-fat cheeses, potato chips, chocolate, and cookies with lower-energy-density options such as fruits, vegetables, and broth-based soups. (These, incidentally, are staples in the Japanese diet ... Judo's birthplace!)

The tactic, or "Judo move," is based on a simple truth: people enjoy eating. And if given the choice between eating more and eating less, they'll almost always choose more. Unlike deprivation-based diets, the Judo-inspired strategy doesn't attempt to fight this natural inclination. By selecting foods with lower energy density, you can eat more—likely even more than you're currently eating—and still weigh less, because you'll be consuming fewer calories.

And here's the good news, supported by solid research: even modest changes in energy density can yield significant benefits.

For example, on a typical day an adult might consume 1200 g of food with an overall energy density of 1.8 kcal/g, giving an energy intake of 2160 kcal. If the average energy density of the diet was decreased by 0.1 kcal/g while the same weight of food was consumed, then the individual would ingest 2040 kcal. Thus, a relatively small change in the overall energy density of the diet would reduce energy intake by 120 kcal per day.[198]

A 120-calorie reduction may seem modest, but it is far from insignificant. As noted earlier, research shows that most people gain weight slowly—just a few pounds per year.[199] Many experts believe that a small energy density reduction, such as a 0.1 kcal/g or roughly 100 kcal per day/is what overweight mitigation efforts need to target. As James Hill, director of the Center for Human Nutrition at the University of Colorado, puts it, "Most of the weight gain seen in the population could be eliminated by some combination of increasing energy expenditure and reducing energy intake by 100 kcal/day."[200]

Hence, the opportunity and reason for optimism: the tweaks to energy density needed to thwart and/or reverse weight gain are modest and entirely achievable for most people. And, therefore, *sustainable.* Indeed, several long-term clinical trials have now confirmed that encouraging people to modestly reduce the energy density of their diets results in sustainable weight loss. Without the deprivation! As one study concluded, "Increasing the amount of food consumed while decreasing energy intake could contribute to the long-term acceptability of a low-energy-dense eating pattern since it could help to control hunger."[201]

Several strategies can reduce the energy density of foods, such as lowering fat and sugar content and increasing the proportion of water-rich fruits and vegetables.[202] I'll walk you through a step-by-step example of how to apply these principles to real-life meal planning. But before we dive into that, it's important to emphasize that increasing water intake isn't limited to solid foods—it *should* also apply to what we drink.

Don't Overlook the Energy Density of what you Drink

When we quench our thirst, we don't just drink water anymore—a zero-calorie affair. Instead, many of us reach for sugary soft drinks. Each 12-oz serving of a carbonated, sweetened soft drink provides about 150 kcal, all from sugar, and offers little to no other nutritional value.[203] These are not only "empty" calories; they are insidiously empty. That's because, experimental results have shown, people do *not* compensate for whatever soft-drink calories they consume when they later sit down for regular meals. As a result, sugary drinks often add energy to our total intake rather than displacing other foods, inevitably leading to increased overall energy consumption.[204]

In a 2007 *Scientific American* article, Barry Popkin, Distinguished Professor of Nutrition and director of the Interdisciplinary Center for Obesity at the University of North Carolina at Chapel Hill School of Public Health, explained how evolutionary history may account for our failure to accurately compensate for liquid calories:

> For most of our evolutionary history, the only beverages humans consumed were breast milk after birth and water after weaning. Because water has no calories, the human body did not evolve to reduce food intake to compensate for beverage consumption. As a result, when people drink any beverage except water their total calorie consumption rises, because they usually continue to eat the same amount of food.[205]

Other researchers have proposed specific physiological mechanisms for this phenomenon.[206] It goes like this: Because liquid meals empty from the stomach more quickly, sensors in the gut have less time to interact with the intake. This shorter exposure weakens the signals that typically indicate fullness and influence meal termination.

This would be merely of academic interest if the beverages humans consumed remained limited to breast milk and water, but increasingly, that is no longer the case.

Market research shows that since the 1970s, soft drink consumption in the U.S. has surged by more than 130 percent (equivalent to an additional 200 calories), outpacing the growth of any other food group.[207] Today, soft drinks account for approximately 10 percent of total energy intake in the American diet (source: CDC's National Health and Nutrition Examination Survey: https://www.cdc.gov/nchs/nhanes/index.htm). This increase in per capita consumption of sugary beverages aligns closely with rising obesity rates.

One reason the rise in soft-drink consumption is a growing concern to those in public health is that the intake rates are even higher among adolescents and children.

> [In the 1970s,] ... the typical teenage boy in the United States drank about seven ounces of soda every day; today he drinks nearly three times that amount, deriving 9 percent of his daily caloric intake from soft drinks. Soda consumption among teenage girls has doubled within the same period, reaching an average of twelve ounces a day... Soft-drink consumption has also become commonplace among American toddlers. About one-fifth of the nation's one- and two-year-olds now drink soda.[208]

A notable 2001 study conducted by the Department of Medicine at Children's Hospital in Boston explored the relationship between childhood soda consumption and obesity.[209] Researchers tracked 548 Massachusetts schoolchildren (average age: 11) over 19 months, monitoring their soda intake and weight changes. The findings were striking: 57 percent of the children increased their soda consumption during the study period, highlighting a concerning trend. The connection between soda consumption and weight gain was so clear-cut that researchers could even link specific amounts of soda to specific amounts of weight gain: each additional daily soda increased a child's BMI by 0.18 points, independent of other dietary factors or exercise.

Perhaps the most surprising finding was that "...the kids were doing something with the soda that few people initially understood: ...[T]hey were not compensating for those extra empty calories when they sat down for regular meals."[210] The clear implication is that sugary drinks add calories without displacing other food intake, leading to an overall increase in energy consumption.[211]

This issue, however, is not unique to children or the U.S. Studies have shown that, like children, adults who consume soft drinks also tend to ingest more total calories than non-consumers.[212] For example, a US study that analyzed seven-day food diaries from 323 adults found that the calories from sugary drinks were added to their overall energy intake without displacing any calories from food."[213] Meanwhile, a Danish study not only confirmed this lack of compensation but also highlighted how quickly increased soft drink consumption can impact weight. In this study, overweight volunteers were given soft drinks sweetened with either sugar or artificial sweeteners and allowed to eat freely. Over the course of ten weeks, those consuming sugared drinks added 500–700 extra calories per day from the beverages alone. Unsurprisingly, they did not compensate for these additional calories and gained an average of 3.5 pounds. What particularly alarmed the Danish researchers was how rapidly these effects occurred.[214]

The takeaway from all this couldn't be clearer: when it comes to quenching thirst, skip the soft drink and reach for water instead.

Now, let's turn our focus to food. While managing solid food intake may not be quite as straightforward, it's entirely doable—as we'll explore next.

"ED-Wise" Meal Selection: A Demo

> *A dieter's worst enemy is staring at a half empty plate and being hungry—and hangry—all the time.*
> Lisa Young,
> Nutritionist, Professor and Author

In Chapter 7, I explain how setting exaggerated weight-loss goals—typically the first or order of business in a weight-loss project—can derail efforts. Poor food selection—our focus here—can do as well.

When it comes to meal planning, most dieters fall victim to what I call the "calories-wise, grams-foolish" trap. After setting their weight-loss goals, they tend to fixate on caloric targets while giving little thought to creating smart, satisfying meals. A common practice, for example, is to simply reduce caloric intake by eating smaller portions of their usual meals, leaving them feeling hungry and deprived. Not exactly a recipe for success. Diets that induce deprivation almost always fail in the long run because they overlook a fundamental truth: people like to eat. A deprived dieter ends up both hungry and unhappy and, before long, they revert to old habits.

But it doesn't have to be this way. The "grams-wise" Judo-esque insight is that by making smarter food choices, a dieter can cut calories *without* triggering hunger. By reducing the energy density of foods, people can eat enough to feel satiated—sometimes even more than before—while still losing weight.

In the remainder of this chapter, I'll demonstrate how to apply this strategy in practice by designing an ED-guided meal plan for a hypothetical dieter: Ms. "X."

Meet Ms. X

Profile:
- Age: 50 years
- Initial Weight: 75 kg (165 lbs.)
- Height: 1.6 meters (5 ft 3 in)
- BMI: 30

Her baseline daily caloric intake—the current level that maintains her at 75 kg weight—is 2,500 kcal/day, distributed as follows:

- Breakfast: 500 kcal
- Lunch: 750 kcal
- Dinner: 1,250 kcal

At a BMI of 30, Ms. X recognizes she is overweight and has decided to go on a diet to lose weight. Her goal is to reduce her daily caloric intake by 20%, bringing it down to 2,000 kcal/day. She hopes this reduction will help her shed about 7.5% of her body weight (5.5 kg, or 12 lbs.) over three months.

This isn't Ms. X's first attempt at dieting. In the past, her go-to strategy was to simply eat less of her usual pre-diet foods—a method that always left her feeling hungry and deprived, and ultimately unsuccessful. (It's no surprise she finds herself back at square one.) This time, she's ready to try something different: a Judo-inspired, ED-driven approach to meal selection that promises to be both satisfying and sustainable.

The task before her now is to design meals that meet her caloric targets while also being enjoyable and satisfying. This means creating meals that deliver not only on quantity (to stave off hunger) but also on quality (to satisfy her preferences). For this demonstration, we'll focus on how she does that for dinner, but she can apply the same procedure for breakfast and lunch.

The first decision she needs to make is how to distribute her 2,000 daily calories among the three meals. This is, of course, a highly personal choice, influenced by lifestyle, family circumstances, and sometimes even culture. For simplicity, we'll assume she decides to retain her pre-diet proportions: 20% to breakfast, 30% to lunch and 50% to dinner. For Ms. X's dinner, this translates to a 1,000-kcal meal.

Generally speaking, composing a 1,000-kcal dinner is no big deal (remember, she used to achieve this by simply cutting her pre-diet portions by 20%.) But that's not her goal here. What she's aiming for now is more ambitious: to design a dinner that not only meets her lower caloric target (1,000 kcal) but is also satisfying—not just in terms of quantity or bulk, but also in terms of quality. Specifically, this means, meals that include only foods *she* enjoys.

Composing such a meal is not only more challenging than simply reducing portion sizes from pre-diet meals, but it's also highly personal. For example, the meal size that satisfies Ms. X may not satisfy you or me. That's why identifying *her preferences* is where she needs to start. While food preferences encompass both quantity and quality, her first priority is to determine the meal size (weight) that satisfies her. Once she establishes *her minimum satiation point*—the smallest portion that meets her needs—she can then proceed to compose the optimal mix of foods that meet her caloric target and any other qualitative preferences or requirements.

Listening to the Gut

We've already learned that the bulk—or weight—of a meal, rather than its energy content, has the overriding influence on satiety—on what makes us feel full. Therefore, the key question for Ms. X (and any potential dieter) is: what dinner *weight* satisfies me? The answer is neither obvious nor universal—it varies from person to person. In fact, I'd argue that understanding this threshold is a vital piece of self-knowledge for anyone striving to maintain or lose weight.

Generally, the meal's "bulk" that satisfies any particular person, tends *not* to be a specific number. Research from Cornell University's Food and Brand Lab[215] suggests that each of us has a narrow weight range for the meals we eat—a "satiation margin"—where we feel content after a meal. If we eat below or above this range, we notice it. But when we eat meals that fall within our satiating range, small variations don't make much difference, and we feel satisfied.

Figuring out one's *satiating margin* (e.g., for a dinner) is relatively straightforward. It requires experimenting with meal sizes that make us feel full and recording their weights. To ensure reliability and confidence in our assessment—and because we're looking for a *range*— it helps to collect multiple data points, such as a week's worth of different meal compositions.

The weight and caloric composition of a dinner meal can be easily assessed using a nutritional database, such as the one provided in the Appendix. These databases list typical portion sizes and include details on macronutrient composition, energy density, calories, and weight. If one's serving size of any food item is larger or smaller, their weight(s) can be determined by physically weighing them using a food scale (Figure 4.4) and then adjusting the caloric content accordingly.

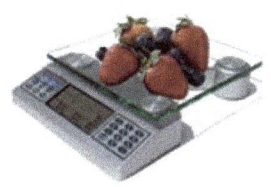

Figure 4.4: Two Options to Determine Food Bulk & caloric content of a meal

The database in the Appendix includes approximately 483 food items, grouped into categories such as "Breads and Grains," "Cereals," "Fruits," "Meat, Poultry and Fish," and more. Each category contains a variety of food items. For example, the "Breads and Grains" category lists 56 items, including bagels, French bread, rye, and sourdoughs. This collection should cover the needs of most readers. However, those seeking a wider range of options may want to explore dedicated nutrition apps. Many of these apps are free to download, with optional in-app subscriptions that offer personalized diet planning, community support, and additional features. One popular app is *Lose It*, which boasts a vast database of nutritional information for millions of foods and even allows users to scan package labels to add new items. Another widely used app is *MyFitnessPal*, which, as of the latest count, includes a database of over 11 million foods.

Back to Ms. X. To begin, she needs to assess her typical pre-diet (maintenance) dinners, which at 1,250 kcal on average, exceed her new caloric target by 250 calories. That said, these pre-diet dinners, have reliably satisfied her hunger.

Using the nutritional database provided in the Appendix, Ms. X can compile and analyze her most recent pre-diet dinner. Figure 4.5 shows an example of what that might look. The energy density (ED), calories, and weights in the table are directly sourced from the Appendix. As shown in the bottom SUM row in Figure 4.5, her dinner's total weight is 650 grams and its total caloric content is 1,226. (The energy density (ED), calories, and weights in the table are directly sourced from the Appendix.) Her dinner's average ED is thus calculated as 1,250 ÷ 650 = 1.9 kcal/gram.

Dinner Entries	ED (cal/g)	Calories	Weight
Cream of mushroom soup, prepared with 2 percent milk	0.79	199.87	253.00
Bread, pita, white	2.75	162.25	59.00
Hummus	1.77	218.60	123.50
Chicken, pieces, boneless, breaded and fried	3.07	325.42	106.00
Potatoes, hash browned	2.18	169.17	77.60
Chocolate chip cookies, homemade	4.88	151.13	31.00
Sum		1226.44	650.10

Figure 4.5: An example of Ms. X's pre-diet dinner

To determine her *satiation margin*, Ms. X needs to repeat this exercise over the course of a week with a variety of dinner compositions. Let's assume she follows through, and after seven dinner experiments, she concludes that the range of dinner sizes that satiate her falls between 600 and 650 grams, with an average weight of 625 grams. The minimum threshold in this range—600 grams—becomes her caloric "line in the sand," representing the minimum amount required for her to feel satisfied after the meal.

Armed with this information, she is now ready to design her optimal meal:

(a) The meal's total *weight* needs to equal or exceed her minimal satiation threshold, with anything between 600 and 650 grams being acceptable.
(b) The meal's total *caloric content* needs to be less than or equal to her target of 1,000 kcal.

This means the average energy density (ED) target for her dinner should be approximately 1.6 kcal/gm, which is 16 % below her current level.

Scouring the Appendix for ideas, she finds a wide variety of options to choose from. Figure 4.6 depicts one of her many satisfying options. Notice that Ms. X cleverly retains a few of her pre-diet favorites (the unshaded entries, such as the hummus). This is a smart move, helping her maintain a sense of normalcy while minimizing feelings of deprivation.

Dinner Entries	ED (cal/g)	Calories	Weight
Lentil and ham soup, canned	0.56	129.75	231.70
Bread, pita, white	2.75	162.25	59.00
Hummus	1.77	218.60	123.50
Chicken breast, roasted, no skin	1.65	135.80	82.30
Potatoes, hash browned	2.18	169.17	77.60
Coffee cake, cinnamon apple, fat-free	2.43	131.35	54.00
Sum		946.92	628.10

Figure 4.6: Satisfying meal

As shown in the bottom SUM row of Figure 4.6, the dinner's total weight is 628 grams—right in the middle of her satiating margin—and its total caloric content of 947, slightly below her target ceiling of 1,000 kcal. Furthermore, it is a meal composed of food items *she* enjoys.

Ms. X has successfully crafted her optimal dinner. *Mission (almost) accomplished!*

Because the database has been expanded to include additional nutritional information—such as macronutrient content—Ms. X can do even more. For instance, she can calculate the breakdown of macronutrients in her optimal meal and assess the caloric contribution of each, as shown in Figure 4.7. And upon inspection make adjustments if desired. (Note: To calculate <u>fat</u> calories, sum the fat grams from all six entries and multiply by 9, since a gram of fat contains approximately 9 kcal. For carbohydrates (CHO) and protein, multiply by 4 kcal/gm.)

Proper nutrient composition is paramount for maximizing energy level, well-being, and overall health. That's why tracking the nutritional composition of our food is always important, but especially so when dieting. While on a diet, we are eating less, putting us at a higher risk of missing out on essential nutrients.

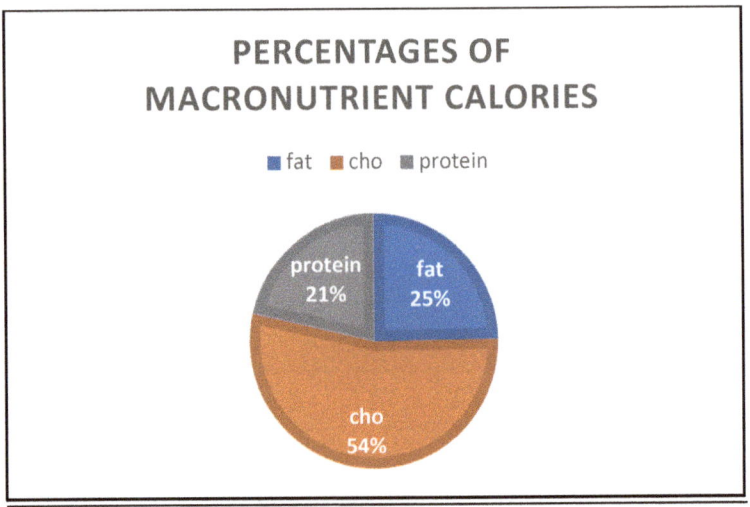

Figure 4.7: Macronutrient composition of Ms. X's optimal meal

By reviewing the macronutrient composition of her selected meal, Ms. X can, if desired, further tweak her meal to meet specific goals. For example, she could adjust the meal to ensure it doesn't exceed fat- or carbohydrate-derived calorie targets or to include a minimum amount of fiber (for health reasons).

Mission accomplished!

Appendix: Nutritional Database

1. Breads and Grain Products

Breads and Grain Products	ED (cal/g)	Calories	Weight	Fat	CHO	Protein	Fiber	Serving Size
Bagel, cinnamon raisin	2.74	197.88	72.22	1.23	39.87	7.08	1.66	1 item
Bagel, plain	2.78	194.60	70.00	1.47	37.10	7.42	1.61	1 item
Biscuit	3.14	88.00	28.00	5.00	10.00	2.00	0.00	1 item
Bread, banana nut	2.01	246.76	123.00	12.15	29.61	3.80	1.14	1.4 oz.
Bread, corn	3.13	169.20	54.00	5.40	26.10	3.60	0.90	1 slice
Bread, French	2.89	72.25	25.00	0.46	14.11	2.94	0.60	1 slice
Bread, hamburger bun	2.82	118.50	42.00	1.80	21.00	4.05	0.00	1 item
Bread, hot dog bun	2.82	118.50	42.00	1.80	21.00	4.05	0.00	1 item
Bread, Italian	2.71	81.30	30.00	1.05	15.00	2.64	0.81	1 slice
Bread, pita, white	2.75	162.25	59.00	0.71	32.86	5.37	1.30	1 item
Bread, pita, whole-wheat	2.66	167.58	63.00	1.64	34.65	6.17	4.66	1 item
Bread, raisin	2.74	109.60	40.00	1.76	20.92	3.16	1.72	1 serving
Bread, rye	2.59	64.75	25.00	0.83	12.08	2.13	1.45	1 slice
Bread, sourdough	2.89	73.87	25.56	0.47	14.43	3.00	0.61	1 slice
Bread, white	2.65	66.25	25.00	0.80	12.27	2.29	0.68	1 slice
Bread, whole-wheat	2.47	61.26	24.80	0.83	10.24	3.21	1.69	1 slice
Bread, zucchini with nuts	3.29	130.57	39.74	7.10	17.03	1.42	0.00	1 slice
Cinnamon roll	3.65	226.12	62.00	10.58	29.18	3.28	1.09	1 item
Couscous, cooked	1.12	89.60	80.00	0.13	18.58	3.03	1.12	1/2 cup
Crackers, cheese	4.89	147.68	30.20	6.87	17.94	3.30	0.69	30 items
Crackers, Nabisco Triscuits, original	4.29	132.86	31.00	4.98	21.04	3.32	3.32	7 items
Crackers, Nabisco Triscuits, reduced fat	3.51	108.92	31.00	2.51	20.11	0.00	3.35	8 items
Crackers, rye crisp bread	3.66	54.90	15.00	0.15	12.30	1.20	2.55	2 items
Crackers, saltine	3.98	110.64	27.80	2.98	18.97	1.98	0.00	10 items
Crackers, saltine, fat free	3.93	109.25	27.80	0.44	22.88	2.92	0.75	10 item
Crackers, wheat	4.56	137.71	30.20	5.24	20.34	2.70	1.12	10 items
Crackers, Wheat Thins, original	4.64	134.64	29.00	4.66	21.75	0.00	1.04	16 items
Crackers, Wheat Thins, reduced fat	4.48	131.21	29.27	4.04	21.20	2.02	2.02	18 items
Croissant, butter	4.06	171.33	42.20	8.86	19.33	3.46	1.10	1 item
Donut, glazed	4.00	242.00	60.50	9.31	32.58	4.65	0.00	1 item
Donut, Jelly	3.18	270.00	85.00	12.00	38.00	4.00	1.00	1 item
Donut, plain, old-fashioned	4.17	196.13	47.00	10.85	21.69	2.71	0.90	1 item
English muffin	2.70	132.30	49.00	0.99	25.80	5.06	1.37	1 item
French toast, with 2 % milk & margarine	2.29	148.39	64.80	7.00	16.20	4.99	0.00	1 slice
Graham crackers	4.23	118.44	28.00	2.83	21.50	1.93	0.78	4 items
Matzo, plain	3.95	110.60	28.00	0.39	23.44	2.80	0.84	1 item
Melba toast	3.64	60.00	16.50	0.48	11.49	1.80	0.90	3 items
Muffin, blueberry	2.93	164.08	56.00	1.82	34.16	1.95	0.78	1 item
Muffin, bran	2.70	155.25	57.50	4.26	27.77	4.03	2.65	1 item
Pancakes, plain	2.33	168.23	72.20	4.93	27.26	3.78	0.72	1 item
Pasta, macaroni, cooked	1.58	111.61	70.70	0.51	21.72	4.04	1.52	1/2 cup

Pasta, noodles, egg, cooked	1.38	112.47	81.50	1.69	20.51	3.70	0.98	1/2 cup
Pasta, spaghetti, cooked	1.57	99.38	63.30	0.59	19.36	3.67	1.14	1/2 cup
Rice, long-grain, brown, cooked	1.11	109.00	98.20	0.88	22.55	2.53	1.77	1/2 cup
Rice, long-grain, white, cooked	1.30	102.96	79.20	0.22	22.31	2.13	0.32	1/2 cup
Rice, pilaf	1.48	138.08	93.30	3.45	23.95	2.74	0.56	1/2 cup
Rice, Spanish	0.88	105.50	120.00	1.82	20.35	2.35	1.35	1/2 cup
Rice, wild, cooked	1.00	83.00	83.00	0.28	17.50	3.25	1.50	1/2 cup
Stuffing, bread	1.77	177.00	100.00	8.60	21.70	3.20	2.90	1/2 cup
Stuffing, cornbread	1.79	179.00	100.00	8.80	21.90	2.90	2.90	1/2 cup
Toaster pastry, fruit	3.91	204.49	52.30	5.52	36.21	2.44	0.58	1 item
Tortilla, corn	2.18	55.59	25.50	0.73	11.38	1.45	1.61	1 item
Tortilla, flour	3.25	112.29	34.55	2.45	19.21	3.01	1.14	1 item
Tortilla, whole-wheat, fat-free	2.00	75.00	37.50	1.00	14.00	3.00	0.00	1 item
Waffle, plain, frozen	2.58	200.00	77.40	6.80	30.00	4.60	1.60	2 items
Waffle, plain, prepared	2.85	213.75	75.00	7.28	32.24	4.85	1.65	1 item

2. Breakfast Cereals

Breakfast Cereals	ED (cal/g)	Calories	Weight	Fat	CHO	Protein	Fiber	Serve Size
100 % Bran, Post	3.67	238.33	65.00	1.08	49.83	8.67	21.67	1 cup
100 % Bran, Post 1/2 cup 1 % milk	1.15	178.17	155.50	2.04	31.92	9.33	10.83	1 cup
100 % Granola, Quaker	4.30	412.00	96.00	####	70.00	10.00	6.00	1 cup
100 % Granola, Quaker 1/2 cup 1 % milk	1.55	265.00	171.00	7.50	42.00	10.00	3.00	1 cup
All-Bran Extra Fiber, Kellogg's	1.92	100.00	52.00	2.00	40.00	6.00	26.00	1 cup
All-Bran Extra Fiber, 1/2 cup1% milk	0.73	109.00	149.00	2.50	27.00	8.00	13.00	1 cup
All-Bran, Kellogg's	2.60	171.60	66.00	3.23	49.00	8.67	19.34	1 cup
All-Bran, Kellogg's with 1/2 cup of 1 % milk	0.91	140.00	154.00	3.50	30.00	9.00	9.00	1 cup
Bite Size Frosted Mini-Wheats, Kellogg's	0.99	146.50	148.50	2.00	28.00	7.50	2.50	1 cup
Bran flakes, Kellogg's	3.17	122.67	38.67	1.33	30.67	4.00	6.67	1 cup
Bran flakes, Kellogg's 1/2 cup of 1 % milk	0.85	120.33	142.33	2.17	22.33	7.00	3.33	1 cup
Bran Flakes, Post	3.20	128.00	40.00	1.33	32.00	4.00	6.67	1 cup
Bran Flakes, Post with 1/2 cup of 1 % milk	0.86	123.00	143.00	2.17	23.00	7.00	3.33	1 cup
Cheerios, General Mills	3.71	110.30	29.73	2.00	21.77	3.59	2.79	1 cup
Cheerios, General Mills 1/2 cup of 1 % milk	0.83	114.15	137.87	2.50	17.89	6.80	1.40	1 cup
Corn Chex, General Mills	3.68	109.22	29.70	0.96	24.91	1.92	0.96	1 cup
Corn Chex, Gen Mills 1/2 cup of 1 % milk	0.82	113.61	137.85	1.98	19.45	5.96	0.48	1 cup
Corn Flakes, Kellogg's	3.57	106.14	29.73	0.12	25.00	2.23	0.98	1 cup
Corn Flakes, Kellogg's 1/2 cup of 1 % milk	0.81	112.07	137.87	1.56	19.50	6.11	0.49	1 cup
Cracklin' Oat Bran, Kellogg's	4.08	298.37	73.10	####	52.21	5.97	7.46	1 cup
Cracklin' Oat Bran, 1/2 cup 1% milk	1.30	208.18	159.55	6.72	33.11	7.98	3.73	1 cup
Crispix, Kellogg's	3.70	118.18	31.94	0.16	27.37	2.14	0.35	1 cup
Crispix, Kellogg's with 1/2 cup of 1 % milk	0.85	118.09	138.97	1.58	20.69	6.07	0.18	1 cup
Golden Crisp, Post	3.90	139.82	35.85	0.47	32.52	2.08	1.00	1 cup
Golden Crisp, Post with 1/2 cup of 1 % milk	0.91	128.91	140.93	1.73	23.26	6.04	0.50	1 cup
Granola, reduced-fat, Healthy Choice	4.20	420.00	100.00	6.00	80.00	10.00	0.00	1 cup
Grape-Nuts Flakes Cereal, Post	3.69	121.77	33.00	1.22	27.03	3.14	3.23	1 cup
Grape-Nuts, Post	3.59	410.34	114.30	2.11	91.55	14.26	10.06	1 cup
Grape-Nuts, Post with 1/2 cup 1 % milk	1.47	264.17	180.15	2.56	52.78	12.13	5.03	1 cup
Honey bunches of oats, Post	3.98	159.20	40.00	2.18	32.48	4.23	1.68	1 cup
Honey bunches of oats,1/2 cup 1% milk	0.97	138.60	143.00	2.59	23.24	6.42	0.84	1 cup
Honey Nut Cheerios, General Mills	3.76	112.80	30.00	1.41	23.97	2.64	2.16	1 cup
Multi Bran Chex, General Mills	3.42	194.94	57.00	1.82	47.14	4.45	7.52	1 cup
Multi Bran Chex, Gen Mills 1/2 cup 1 % milk	1.03	156.47	151.50	2.41	30.57	7.22	3.76	1 cup
Oatmeal, prepared with 1/2 cup of 1 % milk	0.61	147.44	241.70	1.14	32.56	5.00	5.32	1 cup
Oatmeal, prepared with water	0.61	147.44	241.70	1.14	32.56	5.00	5.32	1 cup
Product 19, Kellogg's	3.33	98.90	29.70	0.42	24.65	2.29	0.98	1 cup
Product 19, Kellogg's 1/2 cup of 1 % milk	0.79	108.45	137.85	1.71	19.33	6.14	0.49	1 cup
Puffed Wheat Cereal, Quaker	3.67	44.44	12.12	0.00	8.89	1.62	0.81	1 cup
Raisin Bran, Kellogg's	3.14	172.07	54.80	1.49	42.35	4.23	6.25	1 cup
Raisin Bran, Kellogg's 1/2 cup of 1 % milk	0.96	145.04	150.40	2.25	28.18	7.12	3.12	1 cup
Raisin Bran, Post	3.20	190.08	59.40	1.01	46.39	4.75	8.14	1 cup
Raisin Bran, Post with 1/2 cup 1 % milk	1.01	154.04	152.70	2.00	30.20	7.38	4.07	1 cup
Rice Chex, General Mills	3.75	92.25	24.60	0.34	20.79	1.70	1.08	1 cup
Rice Chex, Gen Mills 1/2 cup of 1 % milk	0.78	105.13	135.30	1.67	17.39	5.85	0.54	1 cup

Rice Krispies, Kellogg's	3.82	142.49	37.30	0.15	33.91	1.60	0.19	1 cup
Rice Krispies, Kellogg's	0.92	130.24	141.65	1.57	23.95	5.80	0.09	1 cup
Shredded Wheat 'n Bran, Post	3.44	189.20	55.00	1.16	45.32	6.00	7.70	1 cup
Shredded Wheat 'n Bran, 1/2 cup 1 % milk	1.02	153.60		2.08	29.66	8.00	3.85	1 cup
Smacks, Kellogg's	3.80	150.86	39.70	0.87	35.13	2.26	1.99	1 cup
Smacks, Kellogg's	0.941	134.43	142.85	1.94	24.57	6.1315	0.993	1 cup
Spoon Size Shredded Wheat, Post	3.51	164.97	47.00	0.99	38.26	5.55	5.83	1 cup
Toasted Oatmeal, original, Quaker	3.88	158.98	41.00	1.67	32.63	4.18	2.51	1 cup
Toasted Oatmeal,1/2 cup of 1 % milk	0.97	138.49	143.50	2.34	23.32	7.09	1.26	1 cup
Toasties, Post	3.60	100.08	27.80	0.03	24.10	1.86	1.25	1 cup
Toasties, Post with 1/2 cup of 1 % milk	0.80	109.04	136.90	1.51	19.05	5.93	0.63	1 cup
Total, General Mills	3.73	148.21	39.70	0.00	34.41	2.65	1.32	1 cup
Total, General Mills with 1/2 cup of 1 % milk	0.93	133.11	142.85	1.50	24.20	6.32	0.66	1 cup
Wheat and barley hot cereal, with water	0.50	122.35	244.00	0.71	27.02	3.89	1.41	1 cup
Wheat Chex, General Mills	3.45	230.12	66.70	1.20	54.83	6.54	8.14	1 cup
Wheat Chex, General Mills 1/2 cup 1 % milk	1.11	174.06	156.35	2.10	34.41	8.27	4.07	1 cup
Wheaties, General Mills	3.53	104.84	29.70	0.68	24.74	2.47	3.00	1 cup
Wheaties, General Mills 1/2 cup of 1 % milk	0.81	111.42	137.85	1.84	19.37	6.23	1.50	1 cup

3. Vegetables

Vegetables	E.D (cal/g)	Calories	Weight	Fat	Carbohy	Protein	Fiber	Serving Size
Alfalfa sprouts	0.24	2.00	8.25	0.00	0.25	0.25	0.25	1/4 cup
Asparagus, boiled, drained	0.22	22.00	100.00	0.22	4.11	2.40	2.00	1/2 cup
Bamboo shoots, canned	0.19	11.40	60.00	0.24	1.93	1.03	0.84	1/2 cup
Beans, green, boiled, drained	0.35	25.55	73.00	0.00	5.84	1.46	2.19	1/2 cup
Beans, green, canned, drained	0.20	13.50	67.50	0.00	3.00	1.00	1.50	1/2 cup
Beans, green, frozen, boiled, drained	0.28	19.00	67.50	0.00	4.50	1.00	2.00	1/2 cup
Beets, boiled, drained	0.44	40.70	92.50	0.17	9.21	1.55	1.85	1/2 cup
Broccoli, boiled, drained	0.35	25.67	73.33	0.30	5.27	1.75	2.42	1/2 cup
Broccoli, raw	0.34	13.60	40.00	0.15	2.66	1.13	1.04	1/2 cup
Brussels sprouts, boiled, drained	0.36	27.00	75.00	0.38	5.33	1.91	1.95	1/2 cup
Cabbage, raw	0.25	15.00	60.00	0.06	3.48	0.77	1.50	1 cup
Carrots, raw	0.41	53.30	130.00	0.31	12.45	1.21	3.64	1 cup
Carrots, sliced, boiled, drained	0.35	24.50	70.00	0.13	5.75	0.53	2.10	1/2 cup
Cauliflower, boiled; drained	0.23	16.10	70.00	0.32	2.88	1.29	1.61	1/2 cup
Cauliflower, raw	0.25	10.83	43.33	0.12	2.15	0.83	0.87	1/2 cup
Celery, raw	0.16	15.20	95.00	0.16	2.82	0.66	1.52	1 cup
Collard greens, boiled, drained	0.33	27.49	83.30	0.60	4.71	2.26	3.33	1/2 cup
Corn on the cob, boiled, drained (medium)	0.94	80.46	85.60	0.63	19.11	2.66	2.40	1 item
Corn, canned, boiled, drained	0.97	80.03	82.50	1.16	17.91	2.76	2.23	1/2 cup
Cucumbers, raw	0.12	16.80	140.00	0.22	3.02	0.83	0.98	1 cup
Eggplant, boiled, drained	0.33	14.29	43.30	0.10	3.52	0.36	1.08	1/2 cup
Fennel bulb, boiled, drained (medium)	0.31	75.33	243.00	0.49	17.74	3.01	7.53	1 item
Green peas, frozen, boiled, drained	0.78	60.45	77.50	0.21	11.05	3.99	4.26	1/2 cup
Green peas, raw	0.81	59.78	73.80	0.30	10.66	4.00	3.76	1/2 cup
Leeks, boiled, drained	0.31	16.43	53.00	0.11	4.04	0.43	0.53	1/2 cup
Lettuce, loose leaf	0.17	8.50	50.00	0.15	1.65	0.62	1.05	1 cup
Lettuce, romaine	0.17	8.50	50.00	0.15	1.65	0.62	1.05	1 cup
Mung bean sprouts, boiled, drained	0.19	12.35	65.00	0.06	2.34	1.32	0.52	1/2 cup
Mushrooms, boiled, drained	0.25	17.50	70.00	0.20	3.56	1.31	1.68	1/2 cup
Mushrooms, raw	0.31	9.30	30.00	0.17	1.53	0.94	0.84	1/2 cup
Okra, boiled, drained	0.22	19.07	86.70	0.18	3.91	1.62	2.17	1/2 cup
Onions, batter-dipped and fried, frozen	4.10	197.00	48.00	11.60	19.20	4.10	1.00	1 item
Onions, chopped, boiled, drained	0.42	48.30	115.00	0.22	10.99	1.56	1.61	1/2 cup
Onions, raw	0.40	15.00	37.50	0.04	3.50	0.41	0.64	1/4 cup
Parsnips, boiled, drained	0.71	55.95	78.80	0.24	13.40	1.04	3.15	1/2 cup
Peppers, green, raw	0.29	19.34	66.70	0.27	4.47	0.53	0.67	1/2 cup
Potato, baked with skin (medium)	0.93	186.00	200.00	0.26	42.30	5.00	4.40	1 item
Potatoes, French-fried	3.33	93.24	28.00	5.24	11.11	0.99	0.90	1 ounce
Potatoes, hash browned	2.18	169.17	77.60	8.92	21.81	2.45	1.55	1/2 cup
Potatoes, mashed with margarine and whole milk	1.13	113.00	100.00	4.20	16.94	1.96	1.50	1/2 cup
Potatoes, scalloped	0.93	108.81	117.00	5.03	14.94	2.48	1.29	1/2 cup
Pumpkin, canned	0.34	47.60	140.00	0.39	11.33	1.54	4.06	1/2 cup
Sauerkraut, canned	0.19	20.90	110.00	0.15	4.71	1.00	3.19	1/2 cup
Spinach, chopped	0.29	10.15	35.00	0.20	1.47	1.27	1.02	1 cup
Squash, summer, boiled, drained	0.20	18.00	90.00	0.28	3.88	0.82	1.26	1/2 cup
Squash, winter, baked	0.40	40.00	100.00	0.09	10.49	0.90	3.20	1/2 cup
Sweet potato, baked	0.92	94.76	103.00	0.15	21.33	2.07	3.40	1/2 cup
Tomato, raw	0.18	23.40	130.00	0.26	5.06	1.14	1.56	1 item
Tomatoes, diced, canned	0.16	20.50	125.00	0.16	4.70	0.95	1.10	1/2 cup
Tomatoes, whole, canned	0.16	20.50	125.00	0.16	4.70	0.95	1.10	1/2 cup
Turnips, boiled, drained	0.22	17.60	80.00	0.06	4.05	0.57	1.60	1/2 cup
Water chestnuts, canned	0.50	35.00	70.00	0.04	8.61	0.62	1.75	1/2 cup

4. Fruit

Fruit	E.D (cal/g)	Calories	Weight	Fat	CHO	Protein	Fiber	Serving Size
Apple	0.52	69.77	135.00	0.00	19.03	0.00	3.62	1 item
Applesauce, unsweetened	0.42	54.60	130.00	0.13	14.65	0.22	1.43	1/2 cup
Apricot	0.48	64.32	134.00	0.52	14.90	1.88	2.68	4 items
Apricots, dried	2.41	78.25	32.50	0.25	20.25	1.00	2.25	1/4 cup
Banana	0.89	107.69	121.00	0.40	27.64	1.32	3.15	1 item
Blueberries	0.57	38.00	66.67	0.22	9.66	0.49	1.60	1/2 cup
Cantaloupe. Cubed	0.34	47.60	140.00	0.27	11.42	1.18	1.26	1 cup
Cherries, sweet	0.63	46.81	74.30	0.15	11.90	0.79	1.56	1/2 cup
Dates	2.82	126.90	45.00	0.18	33.76	1.10	3.60	1/4 cup
Fruit cocktail, in heavy syrup	0.70	91.00	130.00	0.13	24.44	0.61	2.21	1/2 cup
Fruit cocktail, canned in light syrup	0.57	65.55	115.00	0.08	17.17	0.46	1.15	1/2 cup
Grapefruit, pink and red	0.30	36.90	123.00	0.12	9.23	0.68	1.35	1/2 item
Grapes	0.69	90.39	131.00	0.21	23.71	0.94	1.18	1.5 cup
Kiwi fruit, peeled	0.60	45.60	76.00	0.43	10.81	0.93	1.52	1 item
Mango	0.60	46.20	77.00	0.29	11.53	0.63	1.23	1/2 cup
honeydew, cubed	0.36	55.80	155.00	0.22	14.09	0.84	1.24	1 cup
Orange	0.46	57.04	124.00	0.26	14.31	0.87	2.98	1 item
Papaya	0.43	29.03	67.50	0.18	7.30	0.32	1.15	1/2 cup
Peach	0.39	40.95	105.00	0.26	10.02	0.96	1.58	1 item
Peaches, canned in heavy syrup	0.96	136.32	142.00	0.04	37.01	0.67	1.42	1/2 cup
Peaches, canned in light syrup	0.42	54.6	130	0.13	14.43	0.52	1.3	1/2 cup
Pear	0.57	93.08	163.30	0.23	24.87	0.59	5.06	1 item)
Pears, canned in heavy syrup	0.74	95.16	128.60	0.17	24.65	0.26	2.06	1/2 cup
Pears, canned in light syrup	0.47	56.40	120.00	0.12	14.64	0.36	1.92	1/2 cup
Pineapple	0.50	38.00	76.00	0.09	9.97	0.41	1.06	1/2 cup
Pineapple, canned in light syrup	0.52	68.64	132.00	0.16	17.75	0.48	1.06	1/2 cup
Plum	0.46	27.60	60.00	0.17	6.85	0.42	0.84	1 item
Prunes, dried	2.40	102.10	42.50	0.24	27.11	0.98	2.93	1/4 cup
Raisins	3.02	109.63	36.30	0.17	28.87	1.23	1.45	1/4 cup
Raspberries	0.52	31.20	60.00	0.39	7.16	0.72	3.90	1/2 cup
Strawberries	0.32	28.80	90.00	0.27	6.91	0.60	1.80	1/2 cup
Tangerine	0.53	98.05	185.00	0.57	24.68	1.50	3.33	2 items
Watermelon, diced	0.30	48.90	163.00	0.24	12.31	0.99	0.65	1 cup

5. Milk, Yogurt, and Cheese

Milk, Yogurt, and Cheese	ED (cal/g)	Calories	Weight	Fat	CHO	Protein	Fiber	Serving Size
Cheese, American	3.77	105.16	27.90	8.58	2.15	4.29	0.00	1 ounce
Cheese, blue	3.53	100.85	28.57	8.21	0.67	6.11	0.00	1 ounce
Cheese, cheddar	4.03	113.65	28.20	9.35	0.36	7.02	0.00	1 ounce
Cheese, cheddar, reduced-fat	2.86	80.00	28.00	5.00	0.00	9.00	0.00	1 ounce
Cheese, feta	2.64	75.13	28.46	6.06	1.16	4.04	0.00	1 ounce
Cheese, mozzarella, part skim	2.54	71.32	28.08	4.47	0.78	6.81	0.00	1 ounce
Cheese, mozzarella, whole milk	3.00	84.63	28.21	6.30	0.62	6.25	0.00	1 ounce
Cheese, Parmesan, grated	4.31	21.55	5.00	1.43	0.20	1.92	0.00	2 spns
Cheese, provolone	3.51	98.28	28.00	7.45	0.60	7.16	0.00	1 ounce
Cheese, Swiss	3.80	104.99	27.63	7.68	1.49	7.44	0.00	1 ounce
Cottage cheese, fat-free	0.72	82.08	114.00	0.33	7.59	11.79	0.00	1/2 cup
Cottage cheese, full-fat (4 %)	0.98	106.82	109.00	4.69	3.68	12.12	0.00	1/2 cup
Cottage cheese, reduced-fat, 2%	0.86	96.32	112.00	2.74	4.10	13.25	0.00	1/2 cup
Cream cheese, fat-free	1.05	28.67	27.30	0.27	2.09	4.28	0.00	2 spns
Cream cheese, full-fat	3.42	97.81	28.60	9.79	1.16	1.70	0.00	2 spns
Cream cheese, reduced-fat	2.01	56.28	28.00	4.28	2.28	2.20	0.00	2 spns
Cream, half and half	1.30	39.00	30.00	3.30	1.20	0.90	0.00	2 spns
Cream, light	1.95	57.53	29.50	5.70	1.08	0.80	0.00	2 spns
Ice cream, light, vanilla	1.80	118.26	65.70	3.17	19.36	3.14	0.20	1/2 cup
Ice cream, prem, vanilla/choc	2.55	265.20	104.00	17.66	21.58	4.91	0.94	1/2 cup
Milk, low-fat (1 percent)	0.41	104.55	255.00	0.64	14.18	10.10	0.00	8 fl oz.
Milk, nonfat/skim	0.41	88.15	215.00	0.54	11.95	8.51	0.00	8 fl oz.
Milk, reduced fat (2 percent)	0.50	121.00	242.00	4.79	11.62	7.99	0.00	8 fl oz.
Milk, reduced-fat (2%),chocolate	0.71	181.76	256.00	2.56	32.26	8.29	1.28	8 fl oz.
Milk, whole (3.3 percent)	0.61	152.50	250.00	8.13	12.00	7.88	0.00	8 fl oz.
Milk, whole, chocolate	0.80	208.00	260.00	8.50	25.85	7.90	2.00	8 fl oz.
Sour cream, fat-free	0.74	24.66	33.33	0.00	5.20	1.03	0.00	2 spns
Sour cream, full-fat	2.08	62.40	30.00	5.86	1.99	0.72	0.00	2 spns
Sour cream, reduced fat	1.81	54.30	30.00	4.23	2.10	2.10	0.00	2 spns
Yogurt, fat-free, plain	0.59	134.52	228.00	0.89	8.21	23.23	0.00	1 cup
Yogurt, frozen, fat-free, vanilla	1.50	100.00	66.70	0.00	18.00	6.00	0.00	1/2 cup
Yogurt, frozen, fruit flavors	0.95	105.00	110.00	1.35	19.12	4.57	0.00	1/2 cup
Yogurt, fruit-flavors, 99% fat-free	0.95	161.50	170.00	0.34	32.30	7.48	0.00	6 oz.

6. Legumes

Legumes	ED (cal/g)	Calories	Weight	Fat	CHO	Protein	Fiber	Serving Size
Beans, baked, canned	1.05	133.00	126.50	0.50	26.00	6.00	7.00	1/2 cup
Beans, black, canned	0.91	113.75	125.00	0.00	21.25	7.50	8.75	1/2 cup
Beans, lima, boiled, drained	1.23	104.50	85.00	0.50	20.00	6.00	4.50	1/2 cup
Beans, navy, boiled	1.40	127.50	91.00	0.50	24.00	7.50	9.50	1/2 cup
Beans, refried, canned	0.91	108.50	119.00	1.50	18.00	6.50	6.00	1/2 cup
Beans, refried, fat-free, canned	0.79	91.00	115.50	0.50	16.00	6.00	5.50	1/2 cup
Beans, kidney, canned	0.82	106.60	130.00	0.78	18.85	6.79	6.89	1/2 cup
Chickpeas (garbanzo beans), can'd	1.38	164.22	119.00	2.94	27.22	8.38	0.00	1/2 cup
Hummus	1.77	218.60	123.50	10.61	24.85	6.00	4.94	1/2 cup
Lentils, boiled	1.16	111.13	95.80	0.36	19.28	8.64	7.57	1/2 cup
Split peas, boiled	1.18	113.97	96.70	0.39	20.43	8.04	8.04	1/2 cup
Tofu, raw, soft	0.61	70.15	115.00	4.24	2.07	7.53	0.23	4 oz

7. Meat Poultry and Fish

Meat Poultry and Fish	E.D (cal/g)	Calories	Weight	Fat	CHO	Protein	Fiber	Serving Size
Bacon	5.00	70.00	14.00	6.00	0.00	4.50	0.00	2 slices
Beef jerky	4.11	115.00	28.00	7.00	3.00	9.00	1.00	1 ounce
Bologna, beef	2.99	170.43	57.00	14.89	2.45	6.22	0.00	2 slices
Bologna, pork	2.47	112.63	45.60	9.06	0.33	6.98	0.00	2 slices
Bratwurst	2.97	273.24	92.00	24.23	1.84	11.22	0.00	1 item
Chicken breast, fried	2.50	215.00	86.00	8.60	17.20	17.20	0.00	3 oz.
Chicken breast, roasted	1.97	164.50	83.50	6.60	0.00	25.00	0.00	3 oz.
Chicken breast, roasted, no skin	1.65	135.80	82.30	3.29	0.00	25.51	0.00	3 oz.
Chicken liver, simmered	1.67	138.61	83.00	5.40	0.72	20.30	0.00	3 oz.
Chicken wing, meat and skin roasted	2.90	246.50	85.00	16.15	0.00	22.95	0.00	3 oz.
Chicken, boneless, breaded and fried	3.07	325.42	106.00	21.58	15.83	16.88	0.95	6 pc
Fish, battered and fried	2.32	199.64	86.10	10.41	14.19	12.30	0.00	3 oz.
Frankfurter, beef	3.22	142.97	44.40	13.04	1.18	5.19	0.00	1 item
Ground beef, lean, broiled, medium	2.71	231.98	85.60	15.25	0.00	22.04	0.00	3 oz.
Halibut, cooked, dry heat	1.11	94.35	85.00	1.37	0.00	19.16	0.00	3 oz.
Ham, 11 percent fat	1.63	140.18	86.00	7.40	3.29	14.28	1.12	3 oz.
Ham, extra lean, 5 percent fat	1.07	90.95	85.00	3.23	0.43	14.10	0.00	3 oz.
Italian sausage (pork),	3.44	295.84	86.00	23.49	3.67	16.44	0.09	3 oz.
Lamb leg, whole, choice, 1/4" fat	2.67	224.28	84.00	18.14	0.00	14.18	0.00	3 oz.
Orange roughly, cooked, dry heat	1.05	88.37	84.40	0.79	0.00	19.06	0.00	3 oz.
Perch, cooked, dry heat	1.17	96.53	82.50	0.97	0.00	20.51	0.00	3 oz.
Pork chop, center loin, broiled	2.09	180.09	86.00	9.11	0.00	22.26	0.00	3 oz.
Pork rinds, fried	5.51	154.18	28.00	8.86	0.00	17.72	0.00	1 ounce
Salami, beef, cooked	2.61	121.37	46.50	10.32	0.88	5.86	0.00	2 slices
Salmon, pink, cooked, dry heat	1.53	129.59	84.70	4.47	0.00	20.00	0.00	3 oz.
Shrimp, boiled or steamed	1.00	84.00	84.00	1.14	0.00	17.15	0.00	3 oz.
Sirloin steak, lean, broiled	1.83	152.26	83.20	4.82	0.00	25.42	0.00	3 oz.
Swordfish, broiled with margarine	1.72	144.31	83.90	6.65	0.00	19.67	0.00	3 oz.
Tuna, canned in oil	1.98	108.90	55.00	4.52	0.00	16.02	0.00	2 oz.
Tuna, canned in water	1.16	63.80	55.00	0.45	0.00	14.03	0.00	2 oz.
Turkey breast, roasted, no skin	1.55	128.65	83.00	4.80	2.55	17.70	0.00	3 oz.
Turkey tenderloin	1.16	98.66	85.00	0.38	0.00	21.25	0.00	3 oz.
Turkey, breast, ground, 99 % fat-free	1.16	99.82	86.00	1.15	0.00	20.73	0.00	3 oz.
Turkey, ground, lean 7 percent fat	1.52	127.50	84.00	6.75	0.00	15.00	0.00	3 oz.
Veal chop, braised	1.59	131.42	82.50	7.30	0.00	15.33	0.00	3 oz.
Yellowfin tuna, cooked, dry heat	1.30	109.59	84.30	0.50	0.00	24.57	0.00	3 oz.

8. Eggs

Egg	ED (cal/g)	Calories	Weight	Fat	CHO	Protein	Fiber	Serving Size
Egg substitute, liquid	0.84	99.03	117.80	3.75	0.94	14.08	0.00	1/2 cup
Egg, fried	1.96	90.16	46.00	6.83	0.38	6.26	0.00	1 item
Egg, hard-boiled	1.55	75.56	48.75	5.17	0.55	6.13	0.00	1 item
Egg, poached	1.43	71.50	50.00	4.74	0.36	6.26	0.00	1 item
Egg, scrmbl w milk & butter	1.49	170.46	114.40	12.56	1.84	11.43	0.00	1/2 cup

9. Soups

Soups	ED (cal/g)	Calories	Weight	Fat	CHO	Protein	Fiber	Serving Size
Beef broth	0.12	30.00	248.00	0.00	2.00	6.00	0.00	1 cup
Black bean soup, condensed, w water	0.46	106.72	232.00	1.53	17.89	5.61	7.89	1 cup
Chicken broth	0.19	38.00	195.00	1.44	2.88	4.80	0.00	1 cup
Chicken broth, fat-free	0.03	5.00	150.00	0.00	0.00	1.00	0.00	1 cup
Chicken noodle soup, condensed, w water	0.25	62.50	250.00	2.02	7.06	3.02	0.00	1 cup
Chicken, rice, and vegetable soup	0.38	82.50	220.00	2.75	11.00	6.42	1.83	1 cup
Cream of broccoli with cheese soup	0.76	179.87	237.00	11.64	15.87	5.29	0.00	1 cup
Cream of mushroom soup, w 2% milk	0.79	199.87	253.00	13.41	17.20	3.42	1.77	1 cup
Gazpacho soup, canned	0.19	43.70	230.00	0.23	4.14	6.67	0.46	1 cup
Lentil and ham soup, canned	0.56	129.75	231.70	2.60	18.91	8.67	0.00	1 cup
Minestrone soup, condensed, w water	0.34	92.82	273.00	2.84	12.72	4.83	1.09	1 cup
N.E. clam chowder, with water	0.35	83.13	237.50	2.40	11.99	3.68	0.71	1 cup
Onion soup, condensed, with water	0.23	66.70	290.00	2.03	9.48	4.35	0.87	1 cup
Split pea soup with ham	0.75	171.38	228.50	3.98	25.25	9.32	2.06	1 cup
Tomato soup, condensed, w 2% milk	0.55	126.50	230.00	2.99	20.59	5.73	1.38	1 cup
Tomato soup, condensed, w water	0.30	63.75	212.50	0.60	13.96	1.68	1.28	1 cup
Vegetable beef soup	0.31	84.63	273.00	2.07	11.08	6.09	2.18	1 cup
Vegetarian vegetable soup	0.33	79.20	240.00	1.08	14.54	2.64	2.64	1 cup

10. Chips, Pretzels, & Other Snacks

Chips, Pretzels, & Snacks	ED (cal/g)	Calories	Weight	Fat	CHO	Protein	Fiber	Serving Size
Pretzel, soft	3.38	283.92	84.00	2.60	58.29	6.89	1.43	1 item
Chips, potato, fat-free	3.79	106.12	28.00	0.17	23.45	2.70	2.10	1 ounce
Chips, tortilla, corn, fat-free	3.18	89.00	28.00	1.00	18.00	2.00	2.00	1 ounce
Pretzels, hard, salted	3.81	106.68	28.00	0.98	22.18	2.55	0.78	1 ounce
Popcorn, plain, popped	3.87	93.65	24.20	1.10	18.85	3.13	3.51	3 cups
Rice cakes, plain	3.87	103.33	26.70	0.75	21.76	2.19	1.12	3 items
Chips, tortilla, corn, low-fat	4.64	130.00	28.00	4.00	21.00	2.00	2.00	1 ounce
Chips, potato, baked	4.69	131.32	28.00	5.10	19.99	1.40	1.34	1 ounce
Popcorn, caramel	4.31	152.36	35.35	4.52	27.96	1.34	1.84	1 cup
Trail mix	4.62	173.71	37.60	11.05	16.88	5.19	0.00	1/4 cup
Chips, tortilla, white corn	4.89	137.00	28.00	7.00	18.00	2.00	1.00	1 ounce
Popcorn, popped in oil	5.83	157.41	27.00	11.76	12.17	1.97	2.19	3 cups
Chips, potato, regular	5.42	151.76	28.00	10.19	14.23	1.84	1.23	1 ounce
Chips, corn	5.18	145.04	28.00	7.95	17.64	1.69	1.48	1 ounce

11. Mixed Foods

Mixed Foods	ED (cal/g)	Calories	Weight	Fat	CHO	Protein	Fiber	Serving Size
Bean and cheese burrito	2.03	189.00	93.00	6.00	27.50	7.50	0.00	1 item
Beef stew with vegetables	0.99	241.56	244.00	13.49	19.15	10.76	2.20	1 cup
Carrot and raisin salad	1.50	130.88	87.00	4.62	21.56	0.77	1.54	1/2 cup
Cheese pizza, thick crust	2.72	189.58	69.70	7.67	21.61	8.36	0.70	1 slice
Chicken chow mein	0.85	216.75	255.00	7.14	21.14	17.24	2.55	1 cup
Chicken pot pie, frozen	1.98	386.10	195.00	22.33	37.03	9.40	0.00	1 item
Chicken salad	2.32	208.50	90.00	15.75	1.30	14.75	0.35	1/2 cup
Chili con carne with beans, canned	1.07	264.29	247.00	8.57	32.36	14.33	8.15	1 cup
Chili with beans, canned	1.12	145.60	130.00	7.14	15.48	7.42	5.72	1/2 cup
Chili, vegetarian with three beans	0.83	189.23	228.00	0.92	35.08	11.08	9.23	1 cup
Chop suey with beef and pork	1.42	354.81	250.00	15.38	42.31	11.06	0.00	1 cup
Cole slaw	0.78	45.24	58.00	1.51	7.20	0.75	0.87	1/2 cup
Fettuccini Alfredo, frozen	1.85	535.89	290.00	25.36	56.24	20.40	0.00	10 oz.
Hot dog with bun, plain	2.76	267.47	96.80	19.11	14.01	10.19	0.64	1 item
Lasagna with meat	1.35	311.85	231.00	11.37	35.48	16.82	3.93	1 piece
Macaroni and cheese	1.49	211.58	142	9.1022	24.5376	7.952	1.562	3/4 cup
Macaroni salad	1.99	179.00	90.00	9.50	20.50	3.35	1.25	1/2 cup
Meat loaf	1.80	220.00	122.00	13.10	7.00	17.50	0.50	1 srving
Pasta salad, packaged	3.60	900.00	250.00	5.00	180.00	35.00	10.00	3.4 cup
Pizza, thin crust, pepperoni	2.72	375.50	138.00	20.73	30.80	17.77	5.92	1/4 pizza
Pizza, thin crust, sausage, frozen	2.77	421.39	152.00	27.09	34.61	15.05	3.01	1/2 pizza
Pork and beans, canned	1.06	138.00	130.00	1.00	25.00	6.00	7.00	1/2 cup
Potato salad	1.43	174.46	122.00	10.00	13.63	3.27	1.59	1/2 cup
Ravioli, cheese, refrigerated	2.69	235.22	87.50	5.65	35.75	11.29	0.00	1 cup
Spaghetti with meat sauce	1.08	230.54	213.00	2.51	42.10	8.52	3.01	3/4 cup
Taco	2.21	369.09	167.00	20.53	26.64	20.66	0.00	1 item
Three-bean salad	0.80	42.89	53.30	0.00	8.58	1.84	1.84	1 srving
Tuna and noodles	0.95	241.90	254.00	4.54	39.31	12.10	3.02	1 srving
Tuna salad	1.87	187.00	100.00	9.26	9.41	16.04	0.00	1/2 cup
Vegetable burger	1.76	127.00	72.00	4.25	9.50	12.70	3.30	1 item

12. Fast Foods

Fast Foods	ED (cal/g)	Calories	Weight	Fat	CHO	Protein	Fiber	Serving Size
Arby's Horsey Sauce	4.29	60.00	14.00	5.00	3.00	0.00	0.00	0.5 oz
Arby's, barbecue sauce	1.43	20.00	14.00	0.00	5.00	0.00	0.00	0.5 oz.
Arby's, Beef 'n Cheddar Sandwich	2.26	440.00	195.00	21.00	44.00	22.00	2.00	1 order
Arby's, French fries	3.31	245.00	74.00	13.00	31.00	3.00	2.00	1 order
Arby's, roast beef sandwich, regular	2.08	320.00	154.00	13.00	34.00	21.00	2.00	1 order
Burger King, chicken sandwich w mayo	2.42	460.00	190.00	17.00	52.00	25.00	3.00	1 order
Burger King, French Toast Sticks	3.49	394.37	113.00	20.05	46.57	6.78	1.58	1 order
Burger King, onion rings	4.17	396.15	95.00	23.97	41.40	3.67	2.57	1 order
Burger King, Whopper with cheese	2.50	730.00	292.00	44.76	48.76	32.67	2.92	1 order
Church's Chicken potatoes and gravy	0.67	67.31	100.00	1.92	11.54	1.92	0.96	1 order
Church's Chicken, chicken breast	2.02	161.90	80.00	6.67	0.00	23.81	0.00	1 piece
Church's Chicken, chicken leg	2.73	152.88	56.00	9.06	4.88	12.19	0.17	1 piece
Dunkin' Donuts, glazed donut	4.26	194.68	45.70	10.47	23.22	2.38	0.69	1 item
Dunkin' Donuts, jelly-filled donut	3.40	233.24	68.60	12.83	26.75	4.05	0.62	1 item
Hardee's cheeseburger	2.68	329.29	123.00	18.89	25.18	14.04	0.97	1 order
Hardee's French fries	2.96	334.81	113.00	16.04	43.25	3.49	4.19	1 order
Hardee's, coleslaw	1.50	171.50	114.00	10.09	20.18	1.01	2.02	1 order
Hardee's, vanilla shake	1.03	360.00	349.50	20.25	39.00	10.50	0.00	12.3 oz.
Jack in the Box, double cheeseburger	2.82	462.48	164.00	26.54	29.47	26.63	1.48	1 order
Jack in the Box, seasoned curly fries	3.42	424.58	124.00	24.80	45.63	4.96	3.97	1 order
KFC, Chicken breast	3.15	528.89	168.00	34.22	16.59	40.44	0.00	1 piece
KFC, Hot and Spicy Chicken breast	2.63	464.57	177.00	27.69	14.83	37.58	3.96	1 piece
KFC, Original Recipe Chicken breast	2.68	450.24	168.00	27.80	14.23	35.68	0.00	1 piece
KFC, Roast Chicken breast (w skin)	1.93	269.15	139.40	11.80	2.14	39.68	0.00	1 piece
KFC, Roast Chicken breast	1.43	173.30	121.00	4.10	1.03	31.79	0.00	1 piece
Little Caesar's Crazy Bread	2.50	98.25	39.30	2.73	16.38	3.28	0.00	1 piece
Little Caesar's Crazy Sauce	0.40	185.00	464.56	0.00	37.00	0.00	12.33	1 order
Long John Silver's, fish, batter-dipped	2.50	212.50	85.00	12.01	14.78	10.16	0.00	1 piece
McDonald's, apple pie, baked	3.23	247.38	76.50	11.92	33.78	1.99	1.99	1 item
McDonald's, bacon, egg, & cheese	3.04	475.15	156.30	29.34	34.79	21.02	1.41	1 item
McDonald's, Chicken McNuggets	3.02	212.61	70.40	13.95	10.62	11.12	0.00	4 pc
McDonald's, Egg McMuffin	2.28	314.64	138.00	13.33	29.90	18.82	1.52	1 item
McDonald's, Fish Filet tartar & cheese	2.82	631.68	224.00	32.79	59.11	25.22	3.14	1 order
McDonald's, French fries	3.23	218.67	67.70	10.47	28.83	2.31	2.64	1 order
McDonald's, Big Mac	2.57	552.55	215.00	32.16	43.17	25.41	3.44	1 order
McDonald's, Qrtr Pounder w Cheese	2.58	506.45	196.30	27.91	39.16	28.64	2.75	1 order
Pizza Hut, Hand Tossed Pizza, cheese	2.71	279.13	103.00	11.22	32.16	12.29	1.85	1 slice
Pizza Hut, pan pizza, pepperoni	2.91	311.37	107.00	13.98	34.02	12.27	2.14	1 slice
Taco Bell, Big Beef Burrito Supreme	1.89	546.21	289.00	23.26	60.89	23.26	9.25	1 burrito
Taco Bell, Nachos Bell Grande	2.46	757.68	308.00	42.04	71.12	23.38	12.63	1 order
Taco Bell, Steak Fajita Wrap	1.99	445.00	224.00	13.00	54.00	29.00	4.00	1 wrap
Taco Bell, taco salad with salsa	1.70	902.70	531.00	48.69	80.18	35.52	15.93	1 salad
Wendy's, chicken sandwich, breaded	2.19	459.07	210.00	18.56	45.91	29.30	1.95	1 order
Wendy's, chili, small	0.88	205.29	233.00	6.16	21.56	17.45	5.13	8.0 oz.
Wendy's, hamburger, single w everything	1.88	415.64	221.00	19.26	37.51	24.33	2.03	1 order

13. Desserts

Desserts	ED (cal/g)	Calories	Weight	Fat	CHO	Protein	Fiber	Serving Size
Angel food cake	2.58	128.01	49.62	0.40	28.68	2.93	0.74	Slice
Apple pie	3.17	400.00	126.00	19.00	54.00	4.00	3.00	Slice
Apple, baked, unsweetened	0.56	95.03	170.00	0.32	25.34	0.53	4.43	1 item
Banana cream pie	2.69	387.00	144.00	20.00	47.00	6.00	1.00	Slice
Brownie, ready-to-eat	4.66	111.05	23.83	6.93	11.96	1.48	0.48	1 item
Carrot cake with cream cheese frosting	4.20	485.00	115.00	12.00	90.00	5.00	0.00	Slice
Cheesecake	3.21	256.80	80.00	18.00	20.40	4.40	0.32	Slice
Cherry pie	2.60	325.00	125.00	13.75	49.75	2.50	1.00	Slice
Chocolate cake with frosting	3.89	248.96	64.00	12.83	33.82	2.23	1.41	Slice
Chocolate chip cookies	4.93	157.71	32.00	8.00	20.57	1.14	0.00	3 items
Chocolate chip cookies, homemade	4.88	151.13	31.00	8.72	18.41	1.94	0.97	2 items
Chocolate chip cookies, reduced-fat	4.54	140.61	31.00	4.43	23.25	2.21	1.11	3 items
Chocolate crème-filled sandwich cookies	4.68	152.76	32.65	7.00	23.32	2.33	1.17	3 items
Chocolate cupcake, cream-filled	3.74	239.36	64.00	7.39	40.98	2.22	0.64	2 items
Chocolate pudding, 2 % milk	1.11	152.07	137.00	2.82	27.07	4.49	1.10	1/2 cup
Coffee cake with crumb topping	4.18	261.67	62.60	14.59	29.23	4.26	1.25	Slice
Coffee cake, cinnamon apple, fat-free	2.43	131.35	54.00	0.00	29.19	2.92	0.00	Slice
Crème-filled sandwich cookies	4.68	136.47	29.17	6.25	20.84	2.08	1.04	2 items
Crème-filled sandwich cookies, Lo-fat	4.61	133.15	28.90	6.19	19.61	1.03	1.03	2 items
Fruit and juice bar, frozen	0.87	81.56	93.75	0.09	18.94	1.13	0.94	1 item
Fruit chewy cookies (Fig Newtons)	3.60	110.00	30.56	2.50	22.00	0.00	1.00	2 items
Fruit chewy cookies, Fig Newtons fat-free	3.44	100.00	29.03	0.00	23.00	0.00	1.00	2 items
Fruit-flavored frozen pop	0.81	40.50	50.00	0.12	9.84	0.00	0.00	1 item
Fudge bar, frozen	1.67	123.83	74.30	4.42	18.58	2.65	0.44	1 item
Gelatin, fruit-flavored	0.62	82.66	133.33	0.00	18.92	1.63	0.00	1/2 cup
Gelatin, fruit-flavored, sugar-free	0.20	20.00	100.00	0.00	4.22	0.83	0.00	1/2 cup
Graham crackers	4.23	118.44	28.00	2.83	21.50	1.93	0.78	4 items
Granola bar, chewy, chocolate chip	4.31	120.67	28.00	4.76	19.80	2.09	1.40	1 item
Granola bar, chocolate chip, low-fat	3.57	100.00	28.00	3.00	18.00	2.00	1.00	1 item
Granola bar, oats and honey	4.26	178.72	42.00	5.36	30.38	3.57	1.79	2 items
Ice cream, cake cone	4.17	32.94	7.90	0.55	6.24	0.64	0.24	1 item
Italian ice, lemon	1.21	212.62	175.00	0.00	52.34	0.00	0.00	1 item
Peach pie	2.23	264.48	118.60	11.86	39.02	2.25	0.95	Slice
Peanut butter cookies, homemade	4.58	164.42	35.90	8.98	18.70	2.94	0.39	2 items
Pound cake, ready-to-eat	3.88	115.24	29.70	5.91	14.49	1.63	0.15	Slice
Pudding, rice	1.18	128.76	109.40	2.90	21.30	3.87	0.97	1/2 cup
Pumpkin pie	2.04	222.36	109.00	10.14	28.78	4.91	0.00	Slice
Sherbet, all flavors	1.44	136.80	95.00	1.90	28.88	1.05	1.24	1/2 cup
Shortbread cookies	5.02	160.64	32.00	7.71	20.64	1.95	0.58	3 items
Vanilla pudding, prepared with 2%t milk	1.01	142.41	141.00	2.44	26.13	4.15	0.00	1/2 cup
Vanilla wafers	4.41	141.12	32.00	4.86	23.55	1.60	0.61	8 items
White cake with frosting	3.57	236.69	66.30	8.22	37.92	3.58	0.53	Slice

14. Beverages

Beverages	ED (cal/g)	Calories	Weight	Fat	CHO	Protein	Fiber	Serving Size
Apple juice	0.46	114.00	248.00	0.00	28.00	0.00	0.00	8 fl oz.
Apple cider, fermented	0.46	47.00	102.25	0.00	11.54	0.00	0.00	4 fl oz.
Beer	0.45	156.00	348.00	0.00	12.00	0.00	0.00	12 fl oz.
Beer, light	0.31	108.00	348.00	0.00	12.00	0.00	0.00	12 fl oz.
Beer, nonalcoholic	0.19	62.05	320.00	0.00	13.30	0.00	0.00	12 fl oz.
Carrot juice	0.40	98.00	245.00	0.37	22.74	2.33	1.96	8 fl oz.
Champagne	0.70	84.00	120.00	0.00	18.00	0.00	0.00	4 fl oz.
Club soda	0.00	0.00	355.00	0.00	0.00	0.00	0.00	12 fl oz.
Cocoa mix, w water	0.55	136.40	248.00	1.36	28.62	2.28	1.24	8 fl oz.
Coffee	0.08	2.00	25.00	0.05	0.09	0.28	0.00	8 fl oz.
Coffee with 1 cream & sugar	0.12	38.50	320.00	0.00	7.50	0.00	0.00	12 fl oz.
Cognac	2.27	69.00	30.42	0.00	2.00	0.00	0.00	1 fl oz
Cola	0.37	140.60	380.00	0.08	36.33	0.27	0.00	12 fl oz.
Cola, diet	0.00	0.00	340.36	0.00	0.00	0.00	0.00	12 fl oz.
Cranberry juice cocktail	0.54	129.60	240.00	0.24	32.45	0.00	0.00	8 fl oz.
Daiquiri	1.87	224.00	120.00	0.00	8.00	0.00	0.00	4 fl oz.
Eggnog	1.35	329.90	244.30	18.27	32.70	9.62	0.00	8 fl oz.
Fruit punch	0.42	101.85	242.50	0.41	25.32	0.17	0.00	8 fl oz.
Gin	2.31	64.29	27.83	0.00	0.00	0.00	0.00	1 fl oz
Gin and tonic	0.70	150.68	215.00	0.04	13.92	0.04	0.00	7 fl oz.
Ginger ale	0.34	140.42	413.00	0.00	36.22	0.00	0.00	12 fl oz.
Grape juice	0.61	156.77	257.00	0.00	40.48	0.00	0.00	8 fl oz.
Grapefruit juice	0.39	93.60	240.00	0.24	22.08	1.20	0.00	8 fl oz.
Lemonade	0.40	99.00	247.50	0.10	25.79	0.17	0.00	8 fl oz.
Margarita	1.47	180.88	123.00	0.00	43.41	0.00	3.62	4 fl oz.
Milk, soy, plain	0.39	103.00	263.00	4.00	9.00	7.90	3.20	8 fl oz.
Orange juice	0.54	120.96	224.00	0.00	30.04	0.45	0.45	8 fl oz.
Pineapple juice	0.53	116.60	220.00	0.26	28.31	0.79	0.44	8 fl oz.
Root beer	0.41	155.80	380.00	0.00	40.28	0.00	0.00	12 fl oz.
Root beer, diet	0.09	35.00	380.00	0.00	9.00	0.00	0.00	12 fl oz.
Sherry, dry	1.50	180.00	120.00	0.00	13.76	0.24	0.00	4 fl oz.
Soda, cream	0.51	192.78	378.00	0.00	50.27	0.00	0.00	12 fl oz.
Soda, lemon-lime	0.41	150.68	367.50	0.00	38.29	0.33	0.00	12 fl oz.
Soda, lemon-lime, diet	0.00	0.00	367.00	0.00	0.00	0.37	0.00	12 fl oz.
Soda, orange	0.48	171.84	358.00	0.00	44.03	0.00	0.00	12 fl oz.
Soda, orange, diet	0.00	0.00	30.00	0.00	0.00	0.00	0.00	12 fl oz.
Sports beverage	0.26	65.00	250.00	0.00	16.08	0.00	0.00	8 fl oz.
Tap water	0.00	0.00	224.00	0.00	0.00	0.00	0.00	8 fl oz.
Tea, brewed, without sugar	0.01	0.20	20.00	0.00	0.06	0.00	0.00	8 fl oz.
Tea, iced, presweeten w lemon	0.40	160.00	400.00	0.00	40.00	0.00	0.00	12 fl oz.
Vegetable juice	0.19	47.50	250.00	0.23	11.38	1.58	2.00	8 fl oz.
Wine cooler	0.56	134.86	240.00	0.05	15.66	0.15	0.00	8 fl oz.
Wine, red	0.85	103.19	121.40	0.00	3.17	0.08	0.00	4 fl oz.
Wine, white	0.82	99.55	121.40	0.00	3.16	0.08	0.00	4 fl oz.
Whiskey	2.50	70.00	28.00	0.00	0.03	0.00	0.00	1 fl oz

Chapter 5

Managing Energy-In
Part B: *How* we Eat and Drink

Feeding Regulation is More Than Just *Physiology*

It is becoming increasingly clear that human food intake is a complex interplay of biological, psychological, and cultural factors, all orchestrated by the brain.[216] In Chapter 3, we explored the *biological drivers* of feeding regulation, focusing on how the quantity and nutrient composition of our meals trigger neural and hormonal signals. These signals are decoded by the brain's feeding-control center to generate sensations of hunger or satiety.[217] However, as I explained earlier, while biological states of need play a leading role, feeding regulation is far from a solo act.

Over the past fifty years, research has demonstrated that human feeding behavior is a highly complex bio-psychological affair—part reflexive, part reflective. Incoming signals from diverse sources within the body *and external environment* are processed by the brain to stimulate or suppress appetite. In this chapter, we shift our focus to the reflective, psychological dimensions of feeding.

Unlike other species, humans are profoundly influenced by cultural and social cues, which can often override biological signals.[218] For instance, cultural norms determine when meals are served, prompting eating regardless of physiological hunger.[219] Beyond timing, these norms shape expectations about "appropriate" meal size, meal duration, and even what constitutes a meal—factors that influence how much and how quickly we eat. Additionally, health goals and, at times, even moral convictions—such as those driving political hunger strikes—further modulate eating behavior.[220]

An ingenious experiment involving amnesic patients dramatically demonstrates how social influences and visual cues can *override* physiological drives.[221] Researchers investigated what would happen if amnesic patients were served consecutive meals without any memory of the previous one. The results were striking:

> [The] amnesic patients who had no recall of what happened more than a few minutes before consumed a second full lunch and began a third, when each was served a few minutes after the prior meal was cleared away. The lack of memory for having just eaten a culturally appropriate, full meal, along with the presence of food, [was] sufficient to maintain eating.[222]

Once eating begins, the decision to stop is influenced by a different set of factors, and, again, biological states of need do play a role but are not the whole story. Both stomach distension and the food-triggered release of hormones from the gastrointestinal tract send satiety signals to the brain, but these are more like suggestions than commands. A man served his favorite dessert may continue eating well past satiation, while a woman on a diet may stop before her body signals fullness to meet personal aesthetic goals.[223]

Besides personal preferences and goals, cultural and social conventions often shape when and how meals end. Experimental studies have shown that conceptions of an "appropriate" meal—like soup, a sandwich, and a drink for lunch—can strongly influence meal termination. Sociocultural factors also play a major role in food *selection* (what we eat). In fact, to understand what foods someone prefers or consumes, the most revealing question to ask is: *What is your culture or ethnic group?* "There is no other single question that would even approach the informativeness of the answer to this question."[224]

This is not to dismiss hunger as a powerful motivator; it undoubtedly plays a role in feeding. However, in today's modern environment of food abundance, the physiological drive for sustenance often takes a back seat. More and more, the choice of what and how much food to consume is being shaped by conscious human choice, environmental factors, and cultural influence.[225]

In summary, human feeding regulation does not operate as a standalone physiological system. Rather, it is a complex bio-psychological phenomenon with interactions between the physiologic and the behavioral, and between people and their external environment.

Turns out, that's both a problem… and an opportunity.

"We shape our environment, and then our environment shapes us."
Winston Churchill

Churchill's insight—originally a quip about the design of The House of Commons—transcends politics. It aptly describes the reciprocal relationship between humans and their surroundings: we influence the environments we inhabit, and in turn, these environments shape our behaviors, including those that impact our health.[226]

> Man himself may be controlled by his environment, but it is an environment which is almost wholly of his own making… When [we change our] physical or social environment "intentionally" … [we play] two roles: one as a controller, as the designer of a controlling culture, and another as the controlled, as the product of a culture… There is much more to be said about man being guided by the systems of his own creation.[227]

In the realm of health and wellbeing, *environment* is not a monolithic concept but rather a layered construct. It is often conceptualized as a multi-faceted onion, comprising different strata that vary in scale (e.g., micro versus macro) and type (e.g., physical versus social). The number and breadth of these layers depend on the issue being explored and the chosen unit of analysis. For our purposes, a simplified two-layered model—with micro and macro scales—will suffice (Figure 5.1).

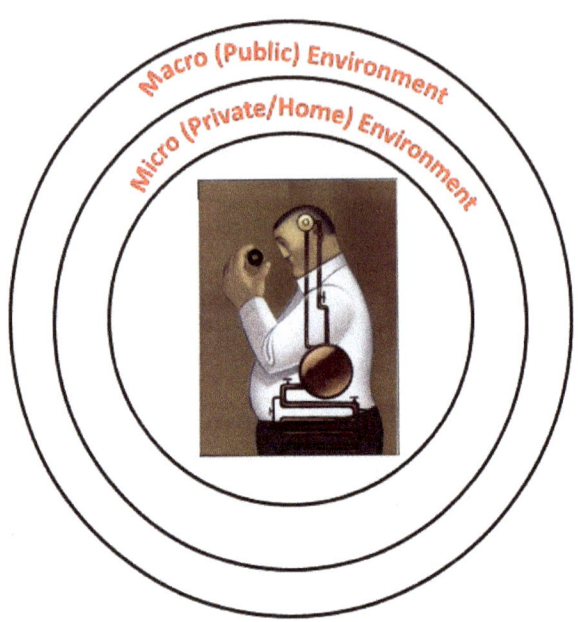

Figure 5.1
Macro and Micro Environments

In this simplified two-tier environmental onion, the outer layer represents the physical and socio-economic macro environment. This encompasses physical aspects, such as the design of our urban setting, alongside socio-economic dimensions, including demographic, technological, political, economic, and cultural factors. It forms the ambient layer that shapes the broad contours of our physical and social landscapes within which we live our lives—what and where we eat and how we work, play, and move about. All of these factors, significantly influence energy intake and expenditure. In a BIG way! How big? In the Appendix to this chapter, I explore how recent, profound shifts in the modern *macro* environment have fueled the obesity epidemic in the United States.

The inner micro-environment circle in Figure 5.1 refers to the immediate surroundings of our homes, which directly influence our daily activities in more intimate ways. This includes physical elements such as the foods and snacks stocked in our pantries, as well as the kitchen and table settings where food is prepared, presented, and served. However, much like the macro environment, this inner layer also encompasses cultural and economic (financial) dimensions. Family environments shape our attitudes, beliefs, and values about food and physical activity. For example, family-instilled values often shape our ideals and aspirations about body weight and shape, which can significantly influence how much energy we strive to consume and expend.

Since the inner layer of the environmental onion is where we can exert the most direct control, it is where we'll focus our attention here. (Macro environmental effects are relegated to the Appendix.) However, before delving into that discussion, it is important to recognize that the two environmental layers are not independent but are deeply interconnected. For example, the foods we choose to eat are not only solely a matter of mom's preferences; they are also shaped by what is available and affordable in our communities—whether in neighborhood restaurants, supermarkets, or vending machines. If nutritious foods are inaccessible or prohibitively expensive, their consumption becomes unrealistic. This makes it misleading—if not outright inaccurate—to suggest that it is simply a person's freely chosen "lifestyle" to stock and eat non-nutritious, high-fat, energy-dense fast foods when healthier options are either much more expensive or altogether unavailable.

Physical factors—such as food availability and accessibility—are not the only ways the micro and macro environments interact. Socioeconomic influences also play a powerful role in shaping our food choices at home. For instance, how food is marketed, distributed, and priced significantly affects what foods people choose to eat. (As will be discussed in the Appendix, when making food choices, individuals often weigh the effect on their wallets as much as the effect on their stomachs.)

While this book focuses on the levers we can directly control to manage our weight and health, we should not forget that we can—and arguably should—wield our clout as citizens and voters to shape public policy and drive changes that transform (or "de-obesify") our macro environment into one that supports healthier living. "Indeed, we can!" And that's not just a political slogan—it's a proven possibility. See sidebar.

> ## Yes, we Can
>
> A few years ago, I witnessed the power of citizen activism firsthand in my hometown of San Francisco. In November 2016, voters in San Francisco—along with those in Oakland and Albany, California—approved ballot measures for soda taxes, driven by growing concern over the rapid rise in obesity rates. The goal was clear: to reduce the consumption of sugar-sweetened beverages like Coca-Cola and Pepsi. These measures were inspired by nearby Berkeley, which had passed a similar tax two years earlier. (Berkeley's early success was later confirmed by a study from the Berkeley Food Institute, which showed that within three years of implementing a penny-per-ounce excise tax on sugar-sweetened beverages, consumption of these drinks had dropped by an impressive 52 percent in the city's low-income and diverse neighborhoods—the very communities suffering the highest rates of diet-related chronic diseases like diabetes and obesity. (https://www.sciencedaily.com/releases/2019/02/190221172056.htm)
>
> This is no isolated case. Bottom-up citizen activism has a long and successful history of shaping public policy and leveraging tools like taxation to discourage the consumption of unhealthful products. Excise taxes on tobacco and alcohol, for example, have been shown to significantly influence consumption patterns.
>
> Clever financial mechanisms, however, don't have to focus solely on discouraging harmful behaviors—they can also incentivize positive ones. Research indicates that subsidies, for instance, can encourage people to consume healthier foods by making them more affordable.

Nonetheless, the closer micro-environment—the home landscape—is the environmental layer over which individuals have immediate and direct control, and thus, the most leverage. As a result, it's also where the rewards are more direct and immediate. This is where our focus now shifts.

The goal of this chapter is to devise practical Judo-inspired home-centered strategies that empower us to control our micro-environment, so it doesn't control us. More specifically, the aim is to create supportive micro-environments that make healthy choices the easy choices.

My set of micro environmental strategies for reshaping *how* we eat falls into three categories. The biological act of swallowing naturally demarcates these three intervention buckets:

- Pre-meal (or pre-swallowing) tactics: Designed to "cue-proof" our feeding environment.
- At-meal tactics: Focused on modulating feeding behavior through the "accelerate-and-brake pedals" that regulate the pace of eating.
- Post-meal (or post-swallowing) tactics: Aimed at managing inter-meal caloric compensation.

Cue-Proofing our Feeding Micro-Environment

We overeat because there are signals and cues around us that tell us to eat.

Brian Wansink[228]

As explained in my discussion of *reward* in Chapter 3, neuroimaging studies suggest that environmental cues signaling palatable foods wield considerable motivational power, often driving us to overeat.[229,230] This applies both to micro-environmental cues in our homes—our focus here—and to macro-environmental ones, such as fast-food advertising.

What makes these cues particularly insidious is their ability to subtly nudge us toward overeating without our conscious awareness.[231] The good news? There's a lot we can do within our homes to mitigate their impact. However, before we can "cue-proof" our feeding environment, we first need to recognize these environmental stimuli. As Peter Senge cautions in *The Fifth Discipline*, "...(environmental) structures of which we are unaware hold us prisoner."[232]

The research of Dr. Brian Wansink—former Executive Director of the USDA's Center for Nutrition Policy and Promotion—and his team at Cornell University's Food and Brand Lab has greatly advanced our understanding of how micro-environmental cues influence our eating behavior. A key insight from their work is that home environments exert a significant—yet often subtle and unconscious—influence on what we eat and how much we consume. To describe these influences, they coined terms like *kitchenscapes* and *tablescapes* to categorize different types of cues within the home.

How powerful are these influences? Wansink's team found that by modifying tablescapes in their lab—using strategies similar to those outlined below—they were able to reduce their subjects' caloric intake by 15% or more. Considering that the average daily caloric intake for American adults is between 2,500 and 3,000 kcal, a 15% reduction is substantial, far exceeding the modest 100 kcal reduction many dieters aim for.

So, how can we apply these laboratory-tested cue-proofing strategies in our own homes? In Wansink's words, it's about *"learning to become illusionists."*[233]

Visual illusions are not just fascinating—they're real and impactful. Examples abound, and some are likely familiar from childhood brain-teaser books or optical illusion puzzles. Let's revisit two text-book examples:

- **Thee Horizontal-Vertical Illusion**
  This illusion resembles an upside-down capital "T" (Figure 5.2). Although the horizontal and vertical lines are exactly the same length, nearly everyone perceives the vertical line as longer—typically by 18–20%. Why? Our brains have a natural tendency to overfocus on the height of objects at the expense of their widths.

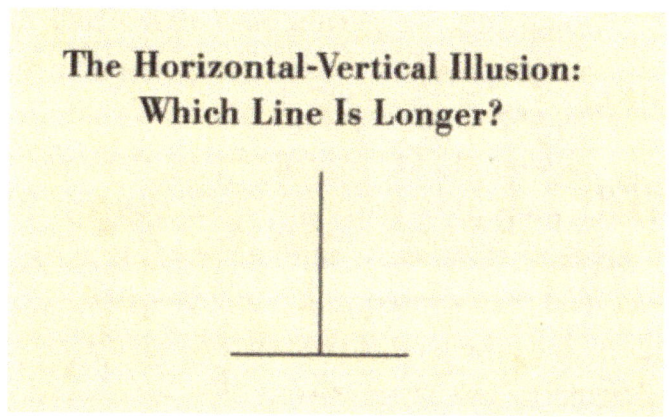

Figure 5.2. Horizontal-vertical illusion

- **The Size-Contrast Illusion**
  Look at the figure below: Which black dot is bigger, the one on the left or the one on the right? The right black dot appears much smaller than the one on the left, even though they are exactly the same size. This happens because we unconsciously use surrounding objects as reference points. For example, in everyday life, a six-foot man standing next to a tricycle seems taller than if he were shown beside a cement truck.

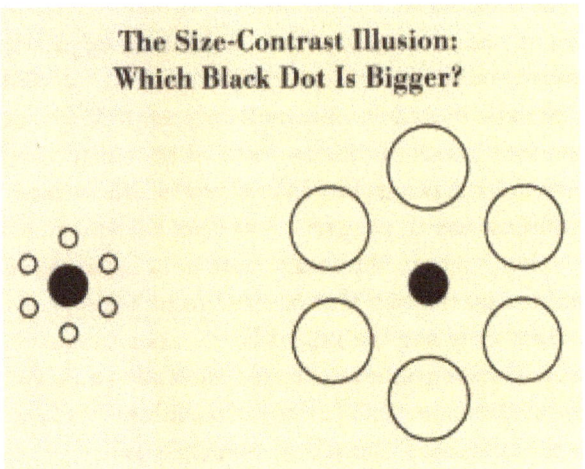

Figure 5.3. Size-contrast illusion

Why is this relevant for us?

Research shows that large containers—such as bowls, plates, and drinking glasses—can create persuasive visual illusions, causing us to misjudge and often underestimate the amount of food or drink they hold. Dito for short wide glass vis-à-vis tall thin glass of the same capacity.

The good news? We can leverage these illusions to our advantage and make them *work for us*.

Cue-proofing the home's feeding landscape

Most of us decide how much to eat before we even take a bite. In a very real sense, we eat "with our eyes." By this, I mean that how food is packaged, presented, and served strongly influences what and how much we consume. For example, visual cues like the size of a popcorn bucket provide subtle yet powerful "suggestions" about how much popcorn to eat. These cues can short-circuit our hunger and satiety signals, leading us to eat beyond satiation.

The menace of the popcorn bucket is no anomaly. Studies on feeding behavior consistently reveal that the shapes and sizes of plates, glasses, and serving dishes convey silent yet powerful cues that shape our expectations about the appropriate portions of food and drinks to serve and eat. Here are some key findings:

- **The size of glasses influences consumption.** Glass size significantly affects how much liquid people perceive is in it—and consequently, how much they consume. For instance, in a "classy" study conducted at the University of Cambridge, researchers found that people drank more wine when it was served in larger glasses. The larger glasses altered participants' perceptions of what constituted a "proper" single serving, causing them to drink faster and consume more overall.[234]
- **Glass shape, not just size, also matters.** Experimental studies have shown that people tend to pour and drink more when using short, wide glasses compared to tall, thin glasses of the same capacity. This effect has been observed across various beverages, including wine, soft drinks, and juice.[235]
- **Larger serving bowls lead to *stealthy* overeating.** Increasing the size of serving bowls can cause dramatic, often unnoticed increases in consumption. In one experiment, participants self-serving snacks from larger (4-quart) bowls took 53% more and ate 59% more than those serving themselves from medium (2-quart) bowls. When questioned about their behavior following the experiment, 87% denied having self-served and eaten differently based on bowl size. Similar experimental results found that when given 34-ounce ice cream bowls versus 17-ounce bowls, people served themselves 31% more ice cream, but did not recognize that they had done so.[236]
- **Serving utensils also matter.** Utensil size and serving method also affect portion sizes. One study found that people given a larger bowl and a larger serving spoon served themselves nearly 60% more ice cream than those with smaller bowls and spoons. Again, participants with the larger utensils were unaware of having taken larger portions.[237]

- **Package size shapes consumption.** When snacking on-the-go or at work, many people eat directly from the package the food comes in, often perceiving the package as a natural consumption unit. Experimental studies show that larger packages lead to increased consumption, regardless of the food's flavor or quality.[238]

How can we turn around the tyranny of *visual illusions* to our advantage? Can we?

Yes, we can. To eat less, we need to take control of our tablescapes—such as the placement and the type of dishes, silverware, drinking glasses, and serving bowls—so that our tablescapes don't control us. This involves managing two key elements: what I call *tablescape hardware* and *tablescape software*. By *hardware*, I mean the physical items such as plates, silverware, drinking glasses, serving bowls, and spoons—stuff you can hold and touch with your hand. *Software*, on the other hand, refers to the rules, habits, and social norms we follow when serving and eating food—such as "mom's rule" about portion size. Just as computer software provides instructions and routines to accomplish a computation or process information, serving software represents the mental codes and conventions we process when making decisions about portions and presentation.

Let's start with *hardware*.

Serving-and-Packaging Hardware

Here are some simple changes we can make in our homes to harness visual cues and make them work *for us,* not against us:

- **Downsize your dinnerware**. Instead of using platter-size dinner plates, opt for smaller, mid-sized plates. Six ounces of goulash on an 8-inch plate looks like a satisfying serving, but the same portion on a 12-inch plate might seem like a mere appetizer. (Interestingly, this downsized approach is standard practice in "Judo Land." In Japan, meals are traditionally served on an array of small plates and bowls rather than one large plate.) Research backs this up: laboratory studies show that moving from a 12-inch to a 10-inch dinner plate leads people to serve and consume 22% less.[239]

- **Shrink your boxes and bowls.** The larger the package you pour from—whether it's cereal at breakfast or cookies while watching TV—the more you'll unconsciously serve yourself. Studies show that oversized packaging can result in consuming 20–30% more.[240] To eat less without sacrificing those supersized savings at the supermarket, consider repackaging jumbo boxes into smaller Ziploc bags or Tupperware containers, and serving them in smaller dishes.
- **"With glasses, think slender if you want to be slender."**[241] Laboratory studies have shown that using tall, skinny glasses instead of short, wide ones causes people—even professional bartenders—to pour less. Up to 30% less.
- **Opt for smaller soda containers.** If soda is your beverage of choice, trade the 20-ounce bottle for a 12-ounce can or, better yet, a mini 7.5-ounce can. (For an even healthier choice, consider switching to water, unsweetened flavored seltzer, or diet soda.)

The Software: "Rebooting" your Serving Routines

Hardware-based interventions have their limitations and may not be sufficient on their own. For example, using a smaller plate or bowl can influence—and often reduce—the amount served and ultimately consumed, but it's not foolproof. This guardrail can still be breached by the over-determined (Figure 5.4.). Besides, when dining out, we obviously have no control over plate size.

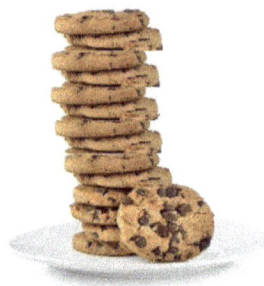

Figure 5.4

Whether at home or eating out, one common "software" error—rooted in our feeding routines—centers on *portion sizes*. Despite its significance, portion size has not received the attention it truly deserves. As I discuss in detail below, this issue is especially pronounced in the U.S., where oversized portions have become the norm. Let's start addressing it here.

Studies consistently highlight two key findings: 1) the portion size served, regardless of plate size, directly impacts food intake; and 2) expanding portion sizes are a growing trend in America. Over the past several decades, portions of many commonly consumed foods—ranging from bagels and muffins to hamburgers and soft drinks—have steadily increased, in sync with the rise in obesity rates. "In particular, this trend has been observed in packaged foods and drinks, as well as energy-dense foods served in the highest-selling take-out establishments, restaurants and fast-food outlets."[242] Today's fast-food portions far surpass those of past generations; in some cases, they are two to five times larger than the servings our parents and grandparents were given in the 1950s and 60s.[243] Consider:

- A typical hamburger in the 1950s weighed 2.8 ounces and contained 200 calories. Today, a typical hamburger weighs 6 ounces and packs 600 calories.[244,245]
- A serving of McDonald's French fries ballooned from 200 calories in the 1960s to 450 calories in the mid-1990s, and now totals 610 calories.[246]

- Beverage sizes have also increased dramatically. "Soft drink containers morphed from eight ounces to twelve ounces to sixteen ounces and then to twenty ounces, as the standard serving size."[247]
- Even cookies have become supersized—with some "monster" cookies today being up to 700% larger than those of several decades ago.[248]

Interestingly, this massive trend of super-sized portions appears to be largely a U.S. phenomenon. When a group of University of Pennsylvania researchers compared restaurant and supermarket meals in the U.S. and France, they found the French portion sizes to be significantly smaller. A soft drink in France is a third smaller, a hotdog 40 percent smaller, and a carton of yoghurt nearly half the size. Even the croissant—perhaps the most iconic French food item—was smaller. A Parisian croissant is a one-ounce affair, while in Pittsburgh, it's twice that.[249,250] It's likely no coincidence that the French are considerably leaner, with an obesity rate of just 15.5 percent—about one-third that of the U.S.

Larger portions obviously create more opportunities for increased caloric intake, but could simply offering bigger servings actually *expand* our appetite? The answer seems to be yes. Experimental studies on humans have established that there is indeed a significant positive association between portion size and energy intake, indicating that we tend to eat more when given larger portions.[251] In other words, "super-sized" and "monster" meals do encourage us to consume more.[252]

In a 2001 study, nutritional researchers led by Barbara Rolls at Penn State University demonstrated that the presence of larger portions *in themselves* "nudged" people toward eating more.

> Men and women volunteers, all reporting the same level of hunger, were served lunch on four separate occasions. In each session, the size of the main entree was increased, from 500 to 625 to 750 and finally to 1000 grams. After four weeks, the pattern became clear: As portions increased, all participants ate increasingly larger amounts, despite their stable hunger levels.[253]

In the experiment, food intake was 30 percent higher when people were given the largest portion compared to the smallest—a significant increase. This led the researchers to confidently conclude that, "human hunger could [indeed] be expanded by merely offering more and bigger options."[254]

But the researchers didn't stop there. Additional studies exploring the underlying mechanisms revealed something both interesting and hopeful for the future: strong cultural influences on our apparent "compulsion" to eat more when served larger portions. These insights emerged from the Rolls group's work with children. The experiments showed that before the age of three, portion size has little impact on a child's energy intake. However, this begins to change between the ages of three and five, as children start to develop and internalize social and cultural conventions regarding food and eating.[255]

In a series of experiments, Dr. Rolls and her colleagues examined the eating habits of two groups of children: one group of three-year-olds and another of five-year-olds.

> Both groups reported equal levels of energy expenditure and hunger. The children were then presented with a series of plates of macaroni and cheese. The first plate was a normal serving built around age-appropriate baseline nutritional needs; the second plate was slightly larger; the third was what we might now call "supersized." The results were both revealing and worrisome. The younger children consistently ate the same baseline amount, leaving more and more food on the plate as the servings grew in size. The five-year-olds acted as if they were from another planet, devouring whatever was put on their plates. Something had happened. As was the case with their adult counterparts . . . the mere presence of larger portions had induced increased eating.[256]

These results suggest that as children grow and develop socially, they shift from eating primarily in response to physiological signals of hunger and satiety—essentially, trusting their gut—to eating in ways that are increasingly influenced by environmental factors, such as portion size, time of day, and social context. The older children had learned that finishing their plate was expected, and that they would be rewarded for doing so.[257]

As children grow into adulthood, they retain the belief that the amount of food served to them is appropriate. As a result, many of us base our decisions about how much to eat in a single sitting on the portion sizes we're given. Indeed, a survey conducted by the American Institute for Cancer Research found that, "67% of those polled said that, when dining out, they finish their entrees most or all of the time."[258] This helps explain why experts believe it's no coincidence that Americans became fatter at the same time they began eating out more and restaurants began super-sizing their portions.[259]

So, while we might like to believe that people stop eating once they feel full, it doesn't work that way. As discussed in more detail in Chapter 3, human appetite, is surprisingly elastic. While this was a useful adaptation in an environment of food scarcity and unpredictability—allowing our hunter-gatherer ancestors to feast whenever food was available and build up fat reserves for future famine—it becomes problematic in our modern environment of food abundance.

Given this, what can we do about large portions?

The answer is simple: *Learn to trim your portions, and you'll trim your calories*. Serving smaller portions may be one of the most effective secrets to eating healthfully and losing weight.

Below are tips and tricks proposed by Lisa Young, adjunct professor of nutrition at New York University (NYU) and author of *Finally Full, Finally Thin: 30 Days to Permanent Weight Loss One Portion at a Time* (Hachette Book Group, 2019), to help you manage your portions while shedding a few pounds along the way:[260]

1. **Institute a half-plate rule**: Follow it at every meal. Better yet, fill half your plate with colorful fruits and vegetables.
2. **Navigating portion control at restaurants**: It might seem challenging, as we don't control the oversized portions typically served. But it needn't be. The proposed tactic: Limit yourself to eating half of what you order and ask for a doggie bag to enjoy the rest on another day.
3. **Guesstimate your portion sizes**: Whether at home, at a restaurant, or snacking on the go, try "palm-sizing!" No one wants to bring

measuring cups and a food scale to dinner, so Dr. Lisa Young offers this simple tip: use your fist to estimate portion sizes (Figure 5.5). For example, a fist-sized portion represents roughly one cup. Want to include meat in your diet without overdoing it? Think of a portion the size of your palm. (Disclosure: I use this "handy" trick every morning at breakfast—I now grab one handful of cereal instead of pouring it directly from the box.)

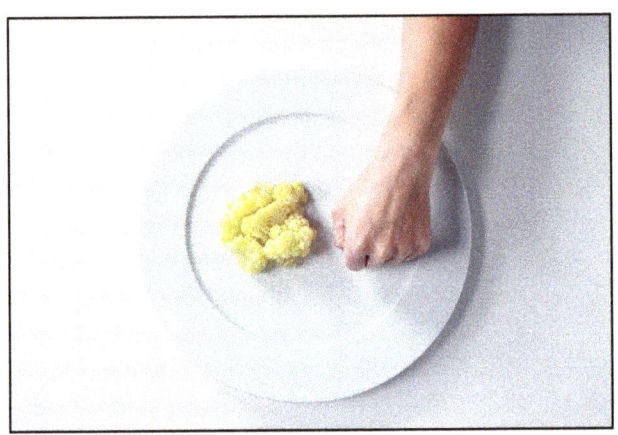

Figure 5.5
A *Judo-esque* tactic to gauge portion size

While surely not a precise instrument—and, of course, hand sizes vary from person to person—using your fist as a rough portion guide can nevertheless be an effective way to manage portion sizes for most meals. Indeed, a recent study from the University of Sydney found that using one's hand to estimate food portions is, in fact, an effective way to assess how much food is on your plate.[261]

At-Meal Tactics: Managing your Accelerate-and-Brake "Feeding Pedals"

The brain relies on gut peptides—such as ghrelin and cholecystokinin (CCK)—to signal how much food has been eaten and the types of nutrients consumed. Like most physiologic processes, these appetite regulatory signals take time to percolate. This means it takes a little while for the body to register that food has reached the stomach and to signal the brain to turn off the feeling of hunger.

Take ghrelin, for example. It's a key peptide hormone secreted when the stomach is empty, triggering sensations of hunger and the urge to eat. As we begin eating, ghrelin levels drop, and we feel less hungry. However, it takes about 20 to 30 minutes for these ghrelin messages to be processed—which is way longer than the blistering eleven minutes the average customer spends eating a meal at McDonald's.[262,263]

By eating too fast—and most Americans do—we tend to over-stuff ourselves before our brains have the chance to apply the "brakes." In 20 to 30 minutes, we can easily wolf down two or three more pieces of pizza and chug a large refill of Pepsi.[264]

Surprise, surprise! This proclivity to rush through meals seems to be most acute in the U.S. According to a global ranking of countries based on mealtime duration published by the OECD, Americans rank near the bottom, spending just one hour a day on mealtimes.

Once again, we can learn from the Japanese. In the OECD study, Japan ranked near the top, with citizens spending a leisurely one hour and 44 minutes each day eating and drinking. The Japanese not only eat smaller portions and use smaller utensils, but they also eat more slowly. There's no "scarfing" down hamburgers and fries in Judo land. Eating with chopsticks helps, as it naturally encourages slower eating with smaller bites. This more leisurely dining style promotes eating less by giving the brain time to signal fullness and may contribute to the fact that the average Japanese consumes 25% fewer calories per day than the average American (*Diets of the World: The Japanese Diet*, WebMD).

OECD's "gold medal," however, goes to the French—they are the top of the league when it comes to leisurely eating. One of the many cliches about France is that mealtimes are sacred, with people spending hours languishing over long meals. The OECD's study backs up this stereotype. According to its findings, the French spend a leisurely two hours, 13 minutes a day drinking and eating. That's the most time spent on meals compared to any other country in the survey, far exceeding the global average of one hour and 30 minutes.

Bottom line: Eating too quickly is a form of *passive* overconsumption. When people eat too fast, they unwittingly consume more.

To mitigate fast-food-induced *passive* overeating, it behooves us to learn from the Japanese and the French and eat more slowly... much more slowly. Rather than wolfing down meals at McDonald's (or at our desks), we would be wise to embrace the French and Japanese tradition—viewing mealtime as a leisurely experience to be savored with friends and family.

In addition to easing off the feeding "accelerator pedal," we must also relearn when to apply the feeding "brake pedal"—that is, when to stop eating.

Relearning when to Apply your "Feeding Brakes"

Among the many practical strategies for mitigating the barrage of environmental pressures to overeat, my favorite is a mealtime principle long practiced by many "leaner cultures:" don't eat until you're hungry, and when you do eat, stop before you feel stuffed.

> Nowadays we think it is normal and right to eat until you are full, but many cultures specifically advise stopping well before that point is reached. The Japanese have a saying—*hara hachi bu*—counseling people to stop eating when they are 80 percent full. The Ayurvedic tradition in India advises eating until you are 75 percent full; [and] the Chinese specify 70 percent. (Note the relatively narrow range specified in all this advice: somewhere between 70 and 80 percent of capacity. Take your pick.) ... That is a completely different way of thinking about satiety. So: Ask yourself not, Am I full? But: Is my hunger gone? That moment will arrive several bites sooner.[265]

The calorie gap between when a Japanese person feels they are no longer hungry and when an American feels they are full is not insignificant. In fact, it's enough to account for the 100 kcal/day reduction that health researchers advocate is needed to eliminate most of the weight gain seen in the population.[266]

Breaking the fast-eating habit is not as straightforward as it may seem, though. It's simply not in our nature to pause after every bite and reflect on whether we're full. Instead,

As we eat, we unknowingly—or mindlessly—look for signals or cues that we've had enough. For instance, if there's nothing remaining on the table, that's a cue that it's time to stop... These cues can short-circuit a person's hunger and taste signals, leading them to eat even if they're not hungry.[267]

What we need to do is the exact opposite: To eat mindfully.

Mindfulness refers to an awareness that arises from paying purposeful attention to the unfolding of an experience—what's referred to in scientific literature as *present-moment awareness*. In this case, the eating experience. Many people associate mindfulness with meditation or exotic Eastern philosophical practices, but it's actually quite simple. Jon Kabat-Zinn, who helped popularize mindfulness in the West, defines it as "paying attention, on purpose, in the present moment, non-judgmentally."[268] Mindfulness is cultivated by learning to purposefully pay attention to present-moment experiences through mindfulness training (MT).

In recent years, several novel mindfulness training interventions, specifically designed to address mindful eating, have been developed.[269] One such tool is an app-delivered mindfulness training program called *Eat Right Now*, developed by Dr. Brewer, an addiction psychiatrist. This app uses mindfulness exercises to help people change their mindless eating habits. And it works. In an empirical assessment of app-based mindfulness training, Brewer et al., (2018)[270] found that these interventions do build mindfulness skills and improve eating habits. However, it takes time. In one study, it took participants at least 10 to 15 tries—and for many, it took 38 or more—to begin reshaping their eating behaviors.[271]

In a recent *New York Times* article titled, "Mindful-Eating Tips that readers shared," (Feb 1, 2022), one piece of advice stood out: *no more multitasking while eating*. Many readers shared their "discovery" that they habitually ate while looking at their phones, reading, working, or watching television. While there's nothing wrong with enjoying food while watching the Super Bowl or during a family movie night, mindful eating is best achieved when your full attention is on the meal.

Post-Meal: Managing Inter-Meal Caloric-Compensation

It is serendipitous that I'm writing this in late November, just before the holiday season—that time of year when many of us subject our bodies to what can only be described as a tsunami of caloric intake. Overeating during the holiday season is a "ritual" familiar to most, and has long been the subject of both popular discussion and academic analysis. For good reason—or is it bad? Recent studies suggest that caloric consumption during the holiday feasts like Thanksgiving and Christmas can increase by 25 to 40 percent.[272] Such significant increases, research findings suggest, "… is a combined result of the eating environment and the food environment. The holiday eating environment directly encourages overconsumption because it involves parties (long eating durations), convenient leftovers (minimal food-prep effort), friends and relatives (eating with others), and a multitude of distractions. At the same time, the food environment—the salience, structure, size, shape, and stockpiles of food—also facilitates overconsumption."[273]

The brief surge in caloric intake during the holidays, in and of itself, isn't necessarily problematic. Rather, the issue lies in people's failure to compensate for the extra intake afterward. This was aptly demonstrated in a two-phase study in which scientists at the National Institutes of Health tracked the amount of weight gained by 195 adults between Thanksgiving and New Year's Day, then checked in with them a year later during phase two. Not surprisingly, the research team found that most of their experimental subjects did gain weight over the holidays. What surprised—and concerned—the researchers, however, was the striking lack of compensation afterward. The inevitable result: the weight gained during the holidays never came off. In fact, 85 percent of the participants (165 out of 195) failed to shed the extra pounds.[274,275] Over time, these small but recurring annual gains gradually accumulate, often leading to chronic obesity.

What explains this failure to compensate? Our own follow-up research suggests a previously underexplored culprit: fundamental ineptitude in "dynamic caloric bookkeeping" (academically referred to as *deficiencies in dynamic reasoning*). As you'll see below, this judgmental deficiency is more widespread than most realize, and its consequences are significant. Misunderstandings about how the *balance*s in the human energy regulation system change over time—as inputs and outputs fluctuate weekly or monthly—can undermine our best efforts to manage weight effectively.

A judgmental deficiency in caloric bookkeeping? That idea surprises most people.

After all, the basics of energy and weight regulation seem relatively straightforward: body weight (and energy stores) change based on the difference between energy intake and expenditure—much like the water level in a bathtub changes depending on the difference between water poured in and water drained out. This process of replenishing and depleting a reservoir—whether it's energy in the body or water in a tub—seems intuitive enough, so it's natural to believe that inferring how such a system behaves dynamically over time—as inputs and outputs fluctuate—should be just as straightforward. Unfortunately, this isn't the case, and it often surprises people.

In the next section, I'll give you an opportunity to "experience" this surprising (and possibly disconcerting) finding firsthand. As the Chinese proverb below suggests, this will not only deepen your appreciation of the cognitive challenge but also offer a more lasting lesson.

Trying your Hand at Inferring Energy and Weight Dynamics

I forget what I hear; I remember what I see; I know what I do.
Chinese proverb

The purpose of this hands-on exercise is to let you assess for yourself the ease—or difficulty—of figuring out how the dynamics of energy and weight balance plays over time, as a function of changes in energy intake and expenditure. You'll also have the opportunity to compare your performance to that of others, including laypeople and healthcare professionals, who tackled the same exercise as part of an experimental study exploring this critical issue.

The study, conceived and led by the author and conducted between 2012 and 2013, aimed to assess people's aptitude for "dynamic caloric bookkeeping." Known as the Systems Inspired Global Obesity Study (SIGOS), its findings were published in the *System Dynamics Review* in January 2014.

This global study was designed to evaluate performance across diverse populations and cultures. Twenty researchers from seven countries—the United States, Venezuela, Norway, France, China, India, and Sri Lanka—participated in the project. To explore whether professional health training improves performance, we sampled two distinct groups: laypeople and healthcare professionals (HCPs). A total of 621 participants took part in the study, 59% of whom were laypeople and 41% healthcare professionals.

The SIGOS Experimental Task—and Your Task Too

We developed a simple task to explore how body weight changes in response to fluctuations in food intake (the inflow) during the holiday season, while keeping daily energy expenditure (the outflow) constant. To make the exercise relatable, we presented participants with a hypothetical overeating scenario, accompanied by a graphical representation of energy intake and expenditure.

As shown in Figure 5.6, Graph (a) depicts the eating behavior of a hypothetical individual during the Thanksgiving-Christmas holiday season. (Look familiar?) In this scenario, the subject initially maintains her weight at 150 lbs., with both daily caloric intake and expenditure at 2,000 kcal. This steady-state situation changes during the holiday periods when her caloric intake increases by 25 percent. Specifically, it is assumed that her food intake rises progressively—and in a linear fashion—peaking at 2,500 kcal/day on Thanksgiving, before tapering back to 2,000 kcal/day. The pattern repeats during Christmas. To simplify the task, expenditure is assumed to remain constant at 2,000 kcal/day throughout.

Given this scenario, our 621 experimental participants—and now *you*—were tasked with sketching on Graph (b) (provided at the bottom of the exercise sheet) how body weight changes over the approximately two-month period. For reference, the initial pre-holiday steady state situation—when body weight was in equilibrium at 150 lbs.—was pre-plotted.

Note to the reader: Before proceeding, take a few minutes to think through the task. Sketch your answer on Graph (b) before moving ahead.

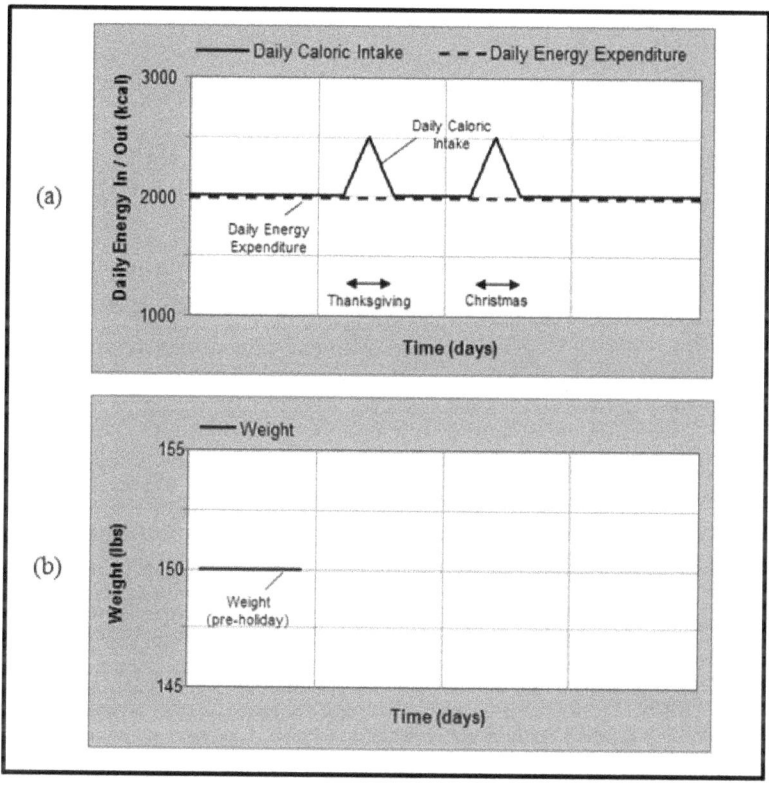

Figure 5.6: The Experimental Task

And the Answer is...

The correct solution to the exercise is provided in Figure 5.8, which is "hidden" on the last page of the chapter (just before the Appendix). If you've already sketched your answer, you may check it now.

A correct solution must exhibit the following two features:

1) It must show that whenever the energy inflow exceeds the (steady) outflow, body weight rises; and

2) Whenever the inflow drops to the level of the outflow (i.e., to 2,000 kcal/day), body weight holds steady.

Obeying these two rules of conservation and accumulation is enough to correctly determine the change in body weight over the two-month stretch. But obeying the rules you must. That's what would allow you, for example, to correctly determine that body weight continues to increase even as energy intake starts to gradually decline right after peaking at 2,500 kcal/day. This is because, although the inflow is decreasing from its peak, it remains higher than the outflow for a few more days—until it reaches the 2,000 kcal level. (For instance, one day after Thanksgiving, food intake may drop from its peak of 2,500 kcal to 2,200 kcal, which would still be 200 kcal greater than the 2,000-kcal energy expenditure level.) And so, as per rule #1, body weight must continue to rise, though at a slowing rate.

Additionally, notice that between Thanksgiving and Christmas, body weight does <u>not</u> return to pre-holiday levels, even though energy intake has returned to its pre-holiday level during this interval. Instead, body weight remains "stuck" at the elevated post-Thanksgiving level. This is because, during this period, energy intake matches energy expenditure (both at 2,000 kcal). When inflow (energy into the body, or water into a bathtub) equals outflow, the total amount in the reservoir (whether our body or a bathtub) *must* remain steady, as per rule #2.

These two rules are all that's needed to describe the changes in body weight accurately. No additional arithmetic is needed.

How did *you* do?

Common Mistakes People Make
If you had difficulty with the task, you are not alone!

In our experiment, many participants struggled as well. Only 24 percent of them got it right. Even more concerning, healthcare professionals (HCPs) performed only slightly better, with 29 percent arriving at the correct answer.

This type of dynamic reasoning experiment has been conducted many times—by me and other researchers—and the results are consistently similar: people tend to underperform. This suggests that inferring the dynamic behavior of even a simple system, such as a single energy reservoir with two flows, may not be as intuitive as we assume.

We also found that in tackling dynamic decision tasks just as this, it is quite common for people to rely on mental short-cuts or "heuristics" to simplify the problem-solving process. This tendency appears to be a fundamental aspect of human nature. These mental shortcuts are often efficient quick-and-dirty strategies that help us reduce mental effort and speed up the process of finding satisfactory solutions—most of the time. Unfortunately, these short-cuts can lead to systematic errors in certain cases. As they do here.

In this task, as well as in many similar ones involving predictions of simple inflow/outflow systems, there is a common tendency to match the shape of the reservoir level (e.g., body weight in our experiment) to the pattern of the inflow. Indeed, in our SIGOS experiment, the majority of those who failed to arrive at the correct answer (and I suspect many readers of this book) sketched a weight trajectory that matched the incorrect pattern shown at the bottom of Figure 5.7 below, where body weight rises and falls in sync with food intake. Did you?

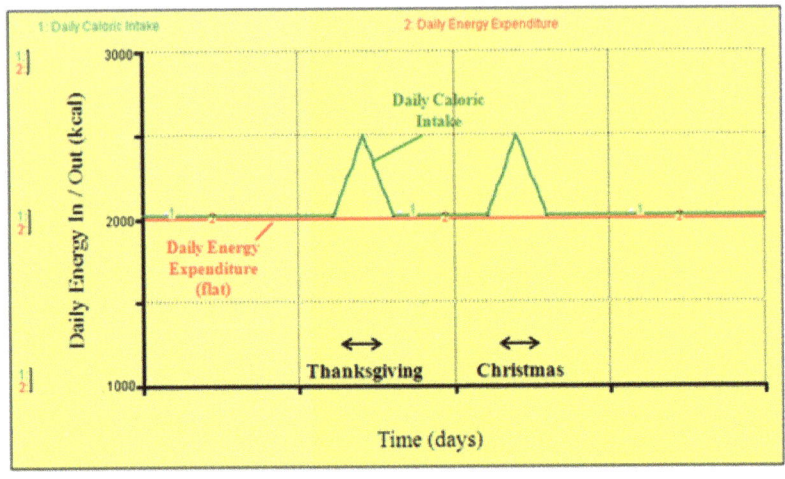

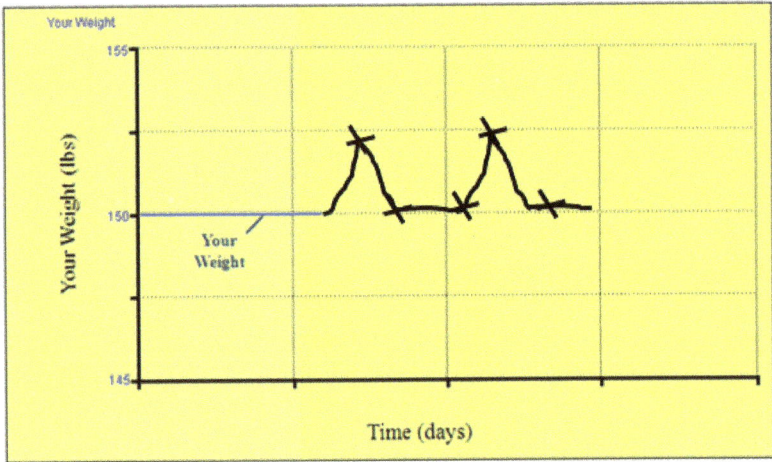

Figure 5.7: Erroneous, but very common pattern-matching response

This so-called "pattern matching" heuristic may seem intuitive, but it is fundamentally flawed. In fact, it violates basic principles of conservation and accumulation in physics. For example, a decline in body weight after the Thanksgiving holiday peak—when energy intake, although declining, is *still* higher than energy expenditure—implies that a reservoir (of energy or matter) is shrinking, even though more is stuff flowing into it than is draining out! This tendency to pattern-match illustrates a basic misconception: that changes in the level of a *reservoir* must directly correlate with changes in the *flow* into it. But this is not the case. The key to whether a reservoir's level increases or decreases is not whether its inflow rate is rising or falling, but rather whether the inflow's magnitude is greater or less than that of the outflow rate. Period! If the inflow is greater, then that would mean more "stuff" is being added to the reservoir than is being drained out. For example, when food intake peaks at 2,500 kcal and starts decreasing to 2,000, body weight should still <u>increase</u> because energy intake, while decreasing, still exceeds energy expenditure.

Another widespread misconception that emerged in our post-experiment interviews—and serves as a RED FLAG for holiday celebrants—is the expectation that after the Christmas festivities, once food intake drops back to its pre-holiday levels, body weight would drop to its original level. It does not. Instead, body weight remains "stuck" at its elevated post-holiday peak! This happens because, after the holidays, energy intake doesn't dip below energy expenditure (as shown in Figure 5.6, Graph [a]). In other words, there is no compensation for the excesses of the preceding months, when energy intake exceeded or equaled outflow but never fell below it.

These findings raise some serious concerns. Most fundamentally: that people can't effectively manage what they don't understand. If individuals misunderstand the basics of inflow/outflow dynamics that underlie human energy regulation, they are likely to make inaccurate assessments of their risk. This, in turn, could seriously undermine efforts to prevent and manage overweight.

Insights and Lessons Learned

The difficulties people encounter with this exercise often come as a surprise. They are surprised because the underlying task—the replenishment and depletion of a reservoir—is a familiar concept, and the experimental scenario is straightforward: energy expenditure is held constant while caloric intake follows a simple pattern (not erratic or chaotic).

Surprise notwithstanding, the results do provide valuable insights. They suggest that caloric bookkeeping might not be as intuitive as we might think, and simple mental shortcuts don't always cut it.

The good news: with just a little training, we can do much better. Specifically, to manage our long-term energy balance and make better inter-meal decisions, we don't need advanced mathematics—just the consistent application of two simple rules:

1) Whenever energy intake exceeds the energy expenditure, body weight increases; and
2) When energy intake equals energy expenditure, body weight remains steady.

Mastering these two simple rules—which govern the replenishment and depletion of our fat reservoir as a function of caloric intake and energy expenditure—can help clear up significant muddles in public thinking about the long-term dynamics of weight gain and loss. And the sooner we grasp these simple concepts of caloric bookkeeping, the sooner we can better regulate the "tap"—before the tub overflows!

Now, let's translate these insights into practical, holiday-specific prescriptions.

Action Plan

First, it's important to recognize that if you overeat during the holidays and then simply return to your pre-holiday routine, your weight will *not* revert to its previous level—it will remain elevated. To shed the added holiday pounds, caloric intake after the holidays must decrease below your normal pre-holiday levels—and by a comparable amount. For example, if you overate by 20% for three days, you should aim to under-eat by 20% for the same duration. Alternatively, you can try to induce a negative energy balance by increasing energy expenditure. However, for most people, this option is usually less appealing—a daily energy deficit of 500 kcal can be achieved by cutting out two cans of soft drinks and a slice of cheesecake, rather than by jogging four miles.

In any case, to effectively compensate for holiday overindulgence, you'll need to accurately estimate the magnitude of the multi-day caloric excess. The good news here is that the cumulative caloric surplus during the holidays is typically not too excessive because it happens over a relatively short period. Nevertheless, it's important to be cautious when assessing caloric intake, as studies consistently show that people tend to underestimate their food consumption—often by as much as 20 to 50%. This is partly because people struggle to remember the details of what they've eaten (especially with the rise in snacking) and because they may feel embarrassed or guilty about recording everything they eat.[276,277]

A possible remedy: keep a food diary to track your daily dietary intake during the holiday period. This will help you more accurately assess the percentage increase in your caloric intake. Since there's a good chance you may overlook a snack or two, it's recommended that you use the higher of two numbers: your assessed percentage increase or a benchmark increase of 33% (which I use). Recall, as noted in studies cited earlier, caloric consumption during Thanksgiving and Christmas increases by 25 to 40 percent. The 33% "safe benchmark" falls in the middle of that range. For instance, if you calculate that over a four-day Christmas gathering, your <u>average</u> caloric intake was 20% above your usual level, you would use the higher 33% figure. It's safer (and healthier) to err on the side of caution.

With that in hand, step two is to devise a plan to compensate. To avoid prematurely dampening the holiday spirit, I recommend an unhurried under-eating plan that works with your body, not against it. Recall from Chapter 4 that research on human satiation suggests each of us has a range for meal size that leaves us feeling content. If we eat significantly less or more than this range, we notice it. But when meals fall within our satiating margin, we feel indifferent to small variations and feel fine. (For most people, the satiating margin is about 20% above or below their usual satiation level.)

To stay within your satiating margin, consider extending your under-eating period to twice or even three times the length of the holiday period. For example, if you overate by 40% over a combined seven-day Thanksgiving/Christmas period, reduce your post-holiday intake by 20% for two weeks instead of cutting it by 40% for one week.

Finally, weighing yourself before and after will help you evaluate your compensation plan and confirm how much weight you've gained and lost. Objective self-monitoring provides valuable feedback, allowing you to track progress, adjust your strategies if needed, and boost your confidence in your self-regulation process by giving you concrete, measurable data. Since weight changes tend to be small, consider investing in a sensitive digital scale, These scales are significantly more precise than traditional dial scales and can detect incremental weight changes as small as a few tenths of a pound.

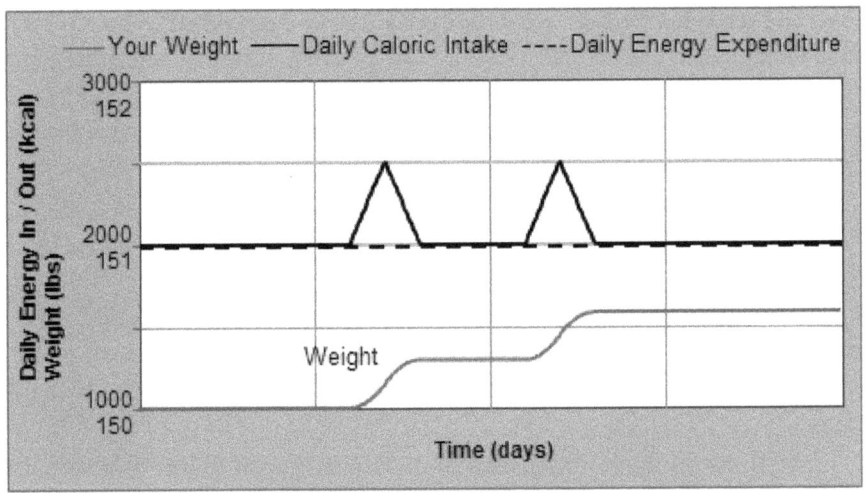

Figure 5.8: The Correct Solution

Appendix

How a Changed Macro Environment Made *US* Fatter

One of the few well-established facts about the obesity epidemic in the US is that it began around the 1980s. According to numerous studies by epidemiologists and public health researchers, its trigger wasn't a single culprit but rather the convergence of multiple socioeconomic and technological shifts that unfolded and reinforced each other in the latter half of the 20th century.

As recently as the 1960s, the primary cost of food—up to 60 percent of its total cost— was the time spent preparing it at home. Back then, most Americans cooked their meals from scratch, using raw agricultural ingredients. However, this began to change in the second half of the century, coinciding with a significant cultural shift: the growing participation of women in the labor force.

In the decades following World War II, the U.S. economy was transitioning from an emphasis on manufacturing to a focus on service industries. Many of the new service-oriented jobs were white-collar roles requiring minimal physical effort. These jobs, often perceived as cleaner and more socially suitable for women than factory work, created new opportunities for female workers. At the same time, women's educational achievements were steadily rising, enabling greater access to interesting and well-paying employment opportunities.

This societal shift created a self-reinforcing cycle. As more women joined the workforce, birth rates declined, reducing the number of years women spent raising young children. This, in turn, freed up more time for career pursuits.[278] By the end of the 20th century, women constituted over 60% of the labor force, a dramatic increase from just 29% in 1950.

This profound evolution in women's roles became one of the most consequential developments shaping America's eating habits over the past 70 years.[279]

As more houschold time was diverted to outside employment, less time and energy were available for home activities such as meal preparation and cleanup.[280] A confluence of technological innovations "greased" these socioeconomic trends, reinforcing the changes in women's lives and reshaping the structure of the American family. Comparable to the mass-production revolution in manufactured goods a century earlier, technological innovations in the preparation, packaging and distribution of food were making it increasingly possible to mass-prepare food, preserve it, and distribute it to consumers in convenient locations for ready consumption.[281,282]

For the growing number of time-strapped, two-earner households, this was a godsend, facilitating a shift from self-prepared meals to mass-prepared options.[283] Postwar prosperity and technological progress thus worked in tandem, creating conditions that accelerated the reallocation of time from housework to outside employment.

With less time to prepare meals, the demand for fast and convenient food surged. The public, perhaps unconsciously, made a tradeoff: sacrificing dietary quality for the sake of convenience and time savings. This shift wasn't driven by a lack of information about the consequences of unhealthy eating but by *incentives*. Even when people know that home-cooked meals are healthier, rational couples may still opt for more convenient, less nutritious options because they prioritize the benefits of their dual-career lifestyles. The high cost of a traditionally cooked meal—in terms of effort, time, or expense—may simply outweigh the perceived health benefits.[284]

The forces driving the demand for convenience in food preparation—namely, the increasing scarcity and growing value of household time—also fueled the long-term trend toward eating out. This trend shows little sign of waning. Today, Americans spend about half of their food budget and consume roughly one-third of their daily calories on meals and drinks consumed outside the home—primarily at the fast-food restaurants that have become ubiquitous across the country since the postwar era.

The growing frequency of convenient, fast-food consumption—both at home and at restaurants—has undeniably contributed to a rise in Americans' average energy intake. Multiple studies examining the relationship between fast-food consumption and increased caloric intake have found that, "fast food restaurant use was positively associated with total energy intake, percent energy from fat, daily servings of soft drinks... and was inversely associated with daily servings of fruit, vegetables, and milk."[285]

The most compelling evidence of this link comes from studies where subjects served as their own controls—comparing their energy intake on days with fast food versus days without it. In one such study, for example, child subjects consumed, on average, an extra 126 kcal per day on days they ate fast food compared to days they did not.[286] Ditto for adults. In a representative study, total energy intake was 40% higher among adult males and 37% higher among females who reported visiting a fast-food restaurant three or more times in the past week, compared to those who reported no fast-food consumption during the same period.[287]

So, what is it about convenience and fast food—whether consumed at home or elsewhere—that induces such a significant increase in caloric consumption? Research suggests three primary mechanisms.

The first is food composition. Like any consumer product, fast food is "designed" for maximum appeal—specifically, to satisfy our primal taste preferences for fats, sugar, and salt.[288] As noted in Chapter 4, eating food rich in fat, the most energy-dense macronutrient, tends to induce *passive overconsumption.* A telling statistic from researchers at the United States Department of Agriculture (USDA) highlights the link between fat-rich fast food and higher caloric intake. They calculate that if fast food had the same average nutritional composition (and thus the same energy and fat density) as home-cooked meals, Americans would consume about 200 fewer calories per day— roughly the equivalent of one extra pound every 20 days.[289]

A second mechanism is America's growing snacking habit. Thanks to the aforementioned technological advances in the preparation, packaging and distribution of convenience food, an enormous variety of tasty, nutrient-poor, high-energy snacks has flooded the U.S. market over the past 50 years—many falling into the nutrient-poor, high energy-dense categories.[290] These are distributed through vending machines that populate workplaces, ensuring that cheap, high-fat, high-calorie snacks are no more than a few steps away.[291] Their increased convenience (and variety), helped fuel a shift in our eating patterns toward frequent "grazing"—small, frequent snacks that accumulate into substantial caloric intake—rather than regular meals. Studies show that, over the last forty years, the amount of energy consumed through snacks has nearly doubled, significantly contributing to an increase in overall energy intake.[292] As Americans began eating more frequently, they ended up eating more overall.[293]

Snacking increases food consumption not only because people are eating more frequently—and often consuming energy-dense foods—but also because snackers typically don't compensate for their snacks by eating less during regular meals.[294,295] In one typical study on snacking, researchers examined the impact of a 400-kcal snack consumed after a 1,300-kcal lunch on subsequent food intake. The snack neither reduced the amount of food consumed at dinner nor delayed the time before the subjects requested dinner.[296] Complementary studies tracking longer-term energy intake support these findings, showing that the total daily energy intake of adult snackers is, on average, 25% higher than that of non-snackers.[297] This suggests that the average adult snacker is effectively eating the equivalent of four full meals a day—rather than three.

There is a third mechanism (alluded to earlier in the chapter): the growing trend toward larger portion sizes, especially when eating out.[298,299] From the restaurants' perspective, the proliferation of Big, Mega, and Super menu items is a profitable and perfectly rational strategy. Compared to the costs of marketing, packaging and labor, the expense of the added ingredients to super-size a menu item is small.[300] While it may cost a restaurant a few pennies to offer 25% more French fries, it can raise its prices substantially more and still offer the consumer a good deal. As a result, these Big, Mega, and Super menu items became a reliable way to boost the average check at restaurants.[301] And because these large portions not only *seem* like bargains, they actually are, consumers love them.

As discussed earlier in the chapter, experimental studies have established a significant positive association between portion size and energy intake, indicating that we eat more when served larger portions.[302] In other words, "super-sized" and "monster" meals induced (and continue to induce) higher caloric intake.[303]

These forces weren't just one-time socioeconomic shocks. Rather—and this is what makes these trends particularly potent—they are *self-reinforcing* processes that continue to grow in a snowballing fashion, feeding on each other and themselves. Instead of causing a single spike in obesity rates, they fuel a trend that continues to escalate.

For example, as the market for convenience food gained momentum, market competition and economies of scale drove relative prices lower. Fat- and sugar-rich foods in the form of snacks, fast foods and beverages became not only convenient and palatable but also incredible bargains relative to other foods. Americans could eat pizza at about a thousand calories a dollar or grab a bag of potato chips or Oreo cookies from a vending machine at around twelve hundred calories a dollar. By comparison—with carrots at 250 calories per dollar, orange juice at 170, and spinach at about 30—fresh foods seemed like a rip-off![304,305]

As the market grew, so did the size and financial power of the major industry players, along with the intensity of market competition. Increases in advertising outlays naturally followed. Today, the U.S. food marketing system ranks as the second-largest advertiser in the economy, after the automobile industry.[306] According to Professor Marion Nestle, chair of the NYU nutrition and food policy department and author of *Food Politics*, food companies spend $33 billion annually advertising and promoting their products—essentially trying to persuade consumers to eat more.[307] And it is working. The massive efforts by food manufacturers and restaurant chains to provide tasty, convenient and affordable foods has led us to consume more calories.[308,309]

Chapter 6

Exercising: Muscling the Body to Work *for us*

First Step: Revisit—and Expand Upon—Common Misconceptions

In Chapter 1, I discussed several entrenched misconceptions about energy and weight regulation—one of the most persistent being the overly simplistic notion that a 3,500-kcal energy deficit equates to a pound of weight loss This overused "magic number" underpins many boilerplate prescriptions in self-help diet and weight-loss books, fueling unrealistic expectations and setting people up for inevitable failures and disappointments.

In reality, losing weight is rarely that straight-forward.

As explained in Chapter 3, when weight is lost, decreases in body weight are accompanied by simultaneous changes in the body's composition (the ratio of fat to lean tissue) and its maintenance energy requirements. These changes, in turn, trigger metabolic adaptations that slow further weight loss until a new energy equilibrium is reached. Overlooking these physio-metabolic complexities often leaves dieters achieving much less weight loss than expected—sometimes dramatically less.

How much less can vary widely from person to person. Overweight individuals are not a homogeneous group—different body types and physiologies respond differently to the same weight-loss intervention. Yet, the crude 3,500-kcal-per-pound formula operates as a one-size-fits-all model, disregarding these individual differences.

Another serious limitation of the simplistic 3,500-kcal-per-pound rule—and one that's central to this chapter—is its inherent limitation to differentiate between various weight-loss strategies. The rule implies, and it is widely held, that a decline in body weight is determined solely by the *size* of the energy deficit, regardless of *how* the energy deficit is induced.

A daily energy deficit, say of 1,000 kcal, can obviously be created in many different ways. For instance, it could be achieved by cutting out four cans of beer and a slice of cheesecake, or by jogging eight miles. Since both strategies produce similar caloric deficits, they are often treated in the media and weight-loss literature—on the back of the 3,500-kcal rule—as being perfectly interchangeable, as if energy were a *single currency*!

It is a significant misconception with serious consequences. For example, it is likely why exercise is so often dismissed as a viable weight-loss option. Rather than investing time and effort into exercise, the misconception of interchangeability understandably steers people toward the easier, quicker, and less costly path of relying solely on dietary restriction. However, since successful weight loss isn't just about losing weight in the short term (and indeed, it shouldn't be), but also about maintaining it over the long term, relying solely on dietary strategies—as we'll see—can be a serious miscalculation.

In this chapter, we will learn that *how* an energy deficit is created does matter. And you'll come to understand that the tradeoff between dieting and exercise is far from *one-dimensional*. Properly assessing this tradeoff requires looking beyond the *quantity* of pounds lost to also include the *quality* of tissue lost—specifically, the FFM/FM composition—and its effects on overall health. Moreover, it's essential to consider both the immediate effects (how much weight is lost in the short term) *and* the long-term sustainability of that loss.

Energy is *Not* a Single Currency

Body weight changes are driven by the balance—or imbalance—between energy intake and energy expenditure. When energy intake matches energy expenditure, body weight remains stable. To lose weight, we need to induce an energy deficit by either reducing energy intake, increasing energy expenditure, or a combination of both.

Whenever we successfully "engineer" an energy deficit and lose weight, we invariably lose both fat mass (FM) and fat-free mass (FFM)—the latter typically comprising muscle mass. This is the fundamental reason why *how* the energy deficit is created matters. The weight-loss strategy we choose to pursue—whether through dieting, exercise, or a combination of both—affects the *composition* of the tissue we lose, i.e., the relative proportions of FM and FFM. And because different tissue types have distinct metabolic characteristics, the composition of the lost tissue not only influences the rate of weight loss but also shapes how the body's energy balance is regulated to maintain the new, lower weight.

Specifically, the metabolic differences between tissue types impact weight-loss dynamics in two primary ways: (1) they determine how much total tissue is shed in the short-term; and (2) they influence how the body's energy requirements change—both during and post weight loss. These metabolic adaptations often persist over time, significantly impacting the long-term prospects for maintaining the weight loss. Moreover, beyond weight loss, differences in the composition of tissue lost inevitably reshape a person's overall body composition, including their overall body-fat percentage. These changes can have significant health implications, which may be either beneficial or detrimental.

In the remainder of this chapter, I will explore these multidimensional effects in more detail and discuss their broader implications for weight loss and overall well-being.

Let's begin by exploring why the composition of lost tissue affects *how much* tissue is lost in the short-term—which is the one (and often only) factor most dieters seem to care about. It is primarily because the energetic density of body mass lost depends on its composition.[310] In other words—and contrary to the 3,500 kcal/lb. rule—the energy cost of losing a pound of body mass is not a fixed 3,500 calories. This figure only represents the energy cost of losing a pound of *pure* fat tissue. Since we typically shed a mix of fat mass (FM) and fat-free mass (FFM) during weight loss, the actual energy cost is almost always different—and often significantly so.

Here is an examination of the metabolic differences between fat mass (FM) and lean body mass (FFM):

> Lean tissue, such as muscle, is about (73%) water, with the remaining (27%) being largely protein with smaller amounts of fat and carbohydrate. In contrast, adipose tissue is only about 15% water, the remainder (85%) being storage lipid with a very small amount of protein contributing to the cell structure and intracellular enzymes. Given these differences in the composition

of body tissues, the amount of energy represented by a (pound) of body weight will differ accordingly. For example, the body energy lost when a (pound) of muscle is lost would be roughly 500 kcal (0.27 * 1,844 kcal/lb. for protein)... Loss of a (pound) of adipose tissue (85% lipid) represents a body energy loss of about 3,500 kcal (0.85 x 4,100 kcal/lb. for pure fat)... Thus, a (pound) of body fat represents nearly (seven) times the energy for fuel represented by a pound of lean tissue.[311]

A striking 7:1 difference in energy density!

With that established, we can now examine how tissue composition affects the *potential* amount of weight lost—before fully accounting for the additional effects of the body's metabolic adaptations—by using a concrete example: a male dieter who has experienced an energy deficit of 1,000 kcal over a 24-hour period.

To illustrate the impact of different tissue compositions in the most intuitive way, let's consider three extreme scenarios: losing only fat mass (FM), losing only fat-free mass (FFM), or losing a 50:50 mixture of the two. (As I will explain below, the actual composition of lost tissue will depend on the type of strategy employed—exercising versus dieting.)

- If our dieter were to lose only FM, he would lose about **0.3 pounds** from an energy deficit of 1,000 kcal (since **1,000 ÷ 3,500 ≈ 0.3**).
- If he were to lose only FFM, he would lose **2 pounds** (since **1,000 ÷ 500 = 2**).
- If he were to lose a 50:50 mix of FM and FFM, he would lose about **half a pound**.

So, as you can see, the differences between the three scenarios are not insignificant. But hold on... these potential short-term projections don't tell the full story.

Next, let's explore why the composition of tissue shed during weight loss affects how much the body's energy requirements change—both during the weight loss process and afterward—and how this, in turn, influences short-term results and long-term weight maintenance. Fundamentally, this is because body composition—the ratio of fat mass

(FM) to fat-free mass (FFM)—is a key determinant of the body's energy needs. Since changes in body composition cause shifts in energy requirements that tend to persist over time, they shape the body's energy profile not just for days or weeks, but for months and even years. As we'll see shortly, this can be a crucial factor in determining long-term success in maintaining weight loss.

The human body, like all systems—whether biological or technological—obeys the laws of thermodynamics, which dictate the immutable principle of energy conservation. Body weight decreases only when energy expenditure exceeds energy intake, and it remains steady when energy-in equals energy-out. This means that successful weight loss requires inducing and sustaining an energy *deficit*, while, maintaining weight loss depends on preserving energy *balance* at the lighter body's new (lower) level of energy expenditure.

And here is the crucial insight: The greater the drop in energy expenditure after weight loss, the harder it will be to maintain the energy balance—and, by extension, the lower weight—over the long term. For example, if your nominal energy expenditure level drops a modest 10% upon losing, say, 50 pounds, your new "normal" daily caloric intake would need to decrease by only 10% compared to your pre-weight-loss diet to sustain your lower weight. That would obviously be more tolerable—and therefore easier to sustain—than if your daily intake had to be cut by 20% or 30% due to a larger drop in your body's energy requirements.

So let us see why the composition of tissue lost—which depends on how weight loss is achieved—affects how much the body's energy requirements change following weight loss, as well as the magnitude of that change.

As you'll recall from Chapter 3, the body's total energy expenditure can be conceptually divided into three components. Approximately 10 percent of daily energy expenditure is expended on processing the food we eat—its digestion and absorption. A second component is the energy expended for muscular work. This typically accounts for 15 to 20 percent of daily energy expenditure but fluctuates as a function of physical exertion. The third and largest component is maintenance energy expenditure (MEE)—also known as basal or resting energy expenditure—which is the maintenance energy required to keep us alive. This is the amount of energy required for essential physiological functions—maintaining cell integrity, body temperature, and vital processes like breathing, heartbeat, red blood cell production, and waste filtration by the kidneys. For most of us the MEE makes up about 60 to 70 percent of total energy expenditure.

How the MEE—by far the largest component of energy expenditure—is distributed among the body's major systems and organs has long been well understood. For example, it is well established that the brain uses more energy than any other human organ, accounting for up to 20 percent of the body's total haul.[312] More recently, research into tissue cellularity and metabolism has provided deeper insights into the metabolic characteristics of the body's two primary tissue types: fat-free mass (FFM) and fat mass (FM). These two compartments exhibit distinct dynamic metabolic profiles, encompassing both qualitative and quantitative differences. What is of significance here is the dynamic differences in energy *consumption* (as opposed to static energy *density*, which was discussed earlier). While fat tissue (primarily inert triglyceride) is relatively inactive metabolically, FFM—such as muscle tissue—has a significantly higher energy-burning rate per unit mass.[313] Empirical studies reveal that the mass-specific metabolic rate of FM (~4 kcal/kg/day) is roughly one-fifth that of FFM (~20 kcal/kg/day). This means each kilogram of lean tissue contributes about five times more to MEE than each kilogram of fat.[314,315]

These stark differences help explain important physiological patterns:[316]

- **Why men typically have higher metabolic rates than women:** Because men generally have more muscle and less fat, which increases their overall energy expenditure.
- **Why metabolic rates decline with age:** Because aging often results in muscle loss, reducing FFM and, consequently, MEE.

So, how does all this relate to our weight-loss maintenance discussion?

When exercise is used to create a desired energy deficit, it tends to protect against the loss of fat-free mass (FFM). This favorable impact on body composition arises primarily from increases in muscle size due to enhanced protein synthesis during exercise. By preserving—or even increasing—FFM, exercise helps blunt the diet-induced decline in metabolic energy expenditure that typically accompanies calorie-restricted weight loss.[317]

Recall from Chapter 1 that a decline in the body's maintenance energy requirements effectively shrinks a diet-induced energy deficit, which unfortunately for the dieter, curbs the rate of weight loss and causes dieters to lose less weight than they expect. Longer-term, as explained above, a persistent decline in MEE in the post-weight-loss state makes it harder to maintain energy balance—and, by extension, to sustain a lower body weight.

Does this necessarily mean then that exercise leads to greater weight loss?

Maybe, maybe not!

The answer to this proverbial "64,000-dollar question" is, unfortunately, far from straightforward. A closer look at our analysis so far reveals why.

On the one hand, exercise can mitigate the decline in MEE—potentially even increase it, if enough muscle mass is added—which could support greater weight loss. On the other hand, because the tissue lost during exercise-based interventions tends to have a higher proportion of fat (which has greater energy density), exercise could result in less weight loss, at least short term. (To remember why, you may want to revisit my hypothetical three-scenario example, comparing the amounts of tissue loss that result from a 1,000-kcal energy deficit, depending on the composition of the lost tissue.)

Answering this question is thus not clear-cut. It requires disentangling conflicting effects of processes that influence body weight in opposing ways—processes that are dynamic and evolve over time. It is a textbook example of what academics refer to as a "dynamically complex computational problem." In this case, one that has been particularly difficult to address due to methodological challenges in field experimentation—such as limitations in conducting studies with sufficiently long durations, large sample sizes, and proper adherence to prescribed exercise protocols.[318]

It's hardly surprising, then, that the answers to our 64,000-dollar question have been inconsistent—even confusing. This has led to increasing recognition of the need to explore alternative methods for testing and experimentation.

Thanks to advances in systems science, biomedical research, and computer technology, we're now equipped to tackle such problems through computer modeling. In addition to being more cost-effective and time-efficient, simulation models enable "perfectly" controlled experimentation. In the model system, unlike the real systems, the effect of changing one factor can be observed while all other factors are held unchanged.[319] Indeed, such computational complex bookkeeping problems are exactly what computer modeling is well-suited to address, and they have been the focus of my own academic training and research.

Over the last decade, I conducted research at Stanford and the Naval Postgraduate School to develop computer models of human physiology for investigating dynamically complex issues related to human and weight energy regulation. Our overarching goal was to create a "virtual laboratory" for exploring the effects of diet and physical activity on body weight and composition. A useful analogy for this kind of model is the flight simulators used by pilots and engineers. Just as a flight simulator mimics an aircraft's behavior in various flight condition, our model simulates human energy and weight regulation in different weight-loss scenarios, offering a platform for researchers to test and analyze the effects of weight-loss strategies in controlled, simulated conditions. (For more on the model's structure and validation, see: Abdel-Hamid, T. (2002). *Modeling the dynamics of human energy regulation and its implications for obesity treatment. System Dynamics Review, 18*(4), 431–471.)

In the remainder of this chapter, I'll briefly discuss an experiment we conducted to compare the effects of physical activity and dietary interventions on body weight and composition, in an attempt to answer our still-unresolved "64,000-dollar question."

The Diet-Exercise Tradeoff... and why 500 kcal ≠ 500 kcal

Simulation-based experimentation has many virtues, but perhaps its most important utility in scientific research is that it makes "perfectly" controlled experimentation possible. These experiments allow researchers to isolate the effects of a single treatment intervention while holding potential confounding variables constant. By systematically conducting a series of such experiments, we can assess and contrast the effects of different treatment options.

Often referred to as the "third branch" of science—alongside theory and experiment—computer simulation has become "...an essential tool in research on problems (ranging) from galaxy formation to protein folding to epidemiology."[320] This includes assessing the efficacy of various health treatment interventions.

Below, I discuss the results of simulation-based experiments in which we sought to compare and quantify the impacts of food restriction versus exercising on both the magnitude and composition of weight loss. (The full study is published in: Abdel-Hamid, T.K. *Exercise and Diet in Obesity Treatment: An Integrative System Dynamics Perspective. Medicine & Science in Sports & Exercise*, 35(3), 400-413.)

The Quantity Dimension

The first issue to settle is the quantity question, that is, assessing and contrasting the changes in body weight—number of pounds or kilograms lost—resulting from calorically-equivalent dieting and exercising interventions. The experimental subjects for this investigation are two overweight sedentary male twins—whom we'll refer to as Mr. "A" and Mr. "B"—with identical initial weights (100 kg) and body compositions (25 percent body fat).

For both individuals, the pre-treatment daily maintenance diet is 14.25 MJ, meaning that a daily caloric intake of 14.25 MJ maintains their bodies at the pre-treatment weight of 100 kg. (Note that in studies of this type, the International System of units is the preferred standard for measuring energy, weight, etc. Food energy is expressed in megajoules (MJ) rather than kilocalories (kcal)—with1 MJ is equivalent to 238 kcal—and body weight expressed in kilograms (kg) rather than pounds, with 1 kg equivalent to 2.2 lbs.)

To compare the impacts of dieting versus exercising, Mr. A is put on a 12-week diet that reduces his daily caloric intake to 12.25 MJ—a drop of 2 MJ (equivalent to 478 kcal). This is compared to the results for Mr. B, who adopts a daily exercise regimen that produces the same caloric deficit of 2 MJ/day. Recognizing that overweight, sedentary individuals are often physically unfit—a limitation that undoubtedly hampers their capacity to exercise—B's daily exercise regimen is stretched over a two-hour period. This allows for a modest exercise intensity level of 1 MJ/hour (which, for example, could be achieved by leisurely walking).

The comparison of changes in body weight over the 12-week period is shown in Figure 6.1. The first thing to notice is that at the end of the three-month intervention, the difference in weight loss between dieting and exercising is quite small. After 12 weeks of dieting, A's body weight drops by 4.9 kg (10.8 lbs.) to 95.1 kg, while a calorically-equivalent daily exercise regimen causes B's weight to drop a comparable 4.7 kg (10.3 lbs.).

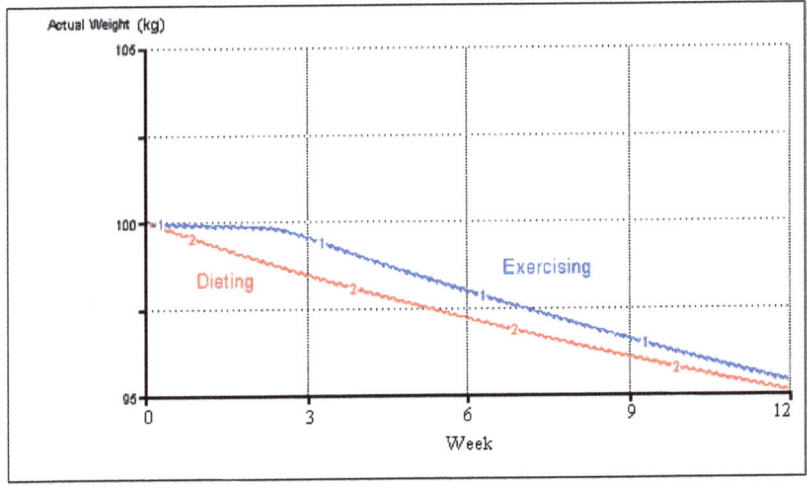

Figure 6.1: Dieting versus exercising

The weight-loss trajectories of the two interventions are quite different, however. With dieting, Mr. A begins losing weight almost immediately, while in the exercise scenario, B's body weight drops very little in the early phases. This flat start in the exercise treatment can be attributed to the increase in muscle size that our sedentary overweight subject enjoys as he embarks on the 2 MJ/day exercise regimen. The initial buildup of B's muscle mass (an addition to his FFM compartment) counterbalances what his body loses in FM, causing a minimal *net* change in total body weight. This exercise effect transitory, however. That's because the gains in muscle mass a person makes when embarking on a new exercise regimen depend on the *relative* intensity of the exercise in comparison to the subject's current fitness level. As Mr. B's fitness improves over time due to sustained exercise at the *same* intensity, this adaptive physiological response—muscle mass gain—eventually levels off.

There is a second dynamic at play. During the first few weeks of an exercise regimen, the body relies on its fat reserves to compensate for both the daily caloric deficit and the initial buildup of muscle mass. While this obviously induces larger losses in FM (in comparison to dieting), it also, perhaps less obviously, precipitates less of a *net* loss in total body mass. Since, as explained earlier, FM has a much larger energy density than FFM, smaller losses in B's FM are used to fuel the buildup of larger gains in FFM. Eventually, though, as the buildup of muscle mass levels off, total weight starts to decline due to the cumulative burden of sustaining a daily energy deficit of two MJ.[321]

The distinctively different trajectories of weight loss from dieting versus exercising have important implications on how people interpret (or misinterpret) treatment outcomes. Consider this: If the duration of the weight-loss treatment were shorter, say four weeks long instead of twelve, Mr. B may conclude, as many probably do, that exercise is an ineffective weight-loss strategy. But that would be both premature and wrong.

In the case of exercise, not only does the magnitude of the caloric deficit matter, but so does duration. Indeed, failure to properly account for this delay effect may help explain why published research results on the efficacy of exercise as a weight-loss intervention have been rather *mixed*. Numerous studies have shown that increased levels of physical activity are as effective as dieting (with some studies showing exercise to be more effective than dieting for long-term weight control). Conversely, an equally large number of studies have reported that exercise has less—or significantly less—effect on weight loss compared to caloric restriction.[322,323] Such mixed findings, not surprisingly, have caused confusion in the public and have led some investigators to discount the importance of exercise in the treatment of obesity.[324]

An American College of Sports Medicine scientific panel review of the issue concluded that the inconsistent results could be attributed, in part, to the complexity and expense of performing longer-term studies, which has often led to most studies being limited to shorter durations.[325] Given that the effects of exercise on body weight typically manifest *after a delay*—as indicated by the findings above—the ACSM emphasized the need for extended-duration studies to fully capture the potential impact of exercise on weight loss.[326] As this study does.

The Composition Dimension

The difference in the time-course of weight loss is not the only distinction between the exercise and diet options. The two treatment strategies also have different impacts on the composition of lost tissue—a distinction that, as I will explain, carries significant long-term implications.

Figure 6.2. shows a comparison of changes in body weight and composition (fat-free mass, fat mass, and percent body fat) between the dieting and exercising strategies. The key finding is that, while the difference in *total* weight-loss is minimal, the difference in tissue composition is significant. As depicted in the figure, during the exercise intervention (represented by the dashed bars), fat mass (FM) drops by 4.2 kg—accounting for nearly 90 percent of the total weight lost—while fat-free mass (FFM) decreases by only 0.5 kg. This contrasts with the diet intervention, where 70 percent of A's weight loss was FM and 30 percent was FFM (with FM dropping by 3.4 kg and FFM losing 1.5 kg).[327]

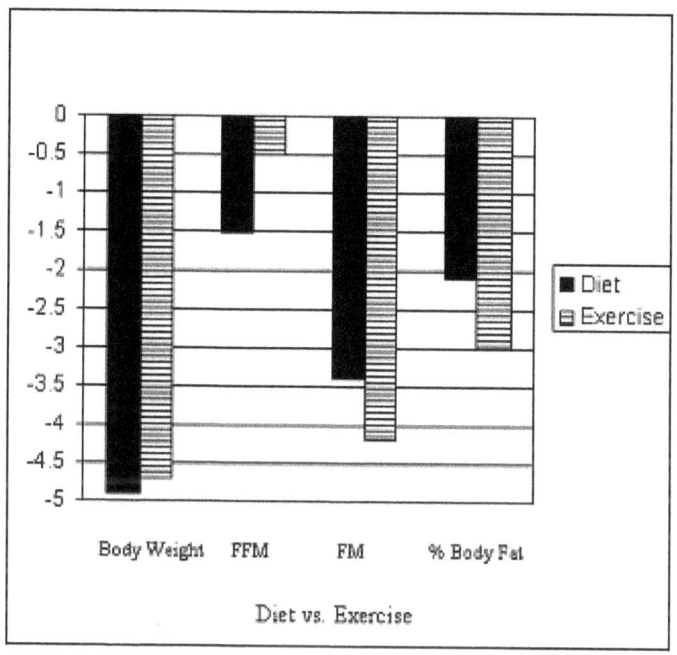

Figure 6.2: Comparing changes to body weight and composition

These differences in tissue composition are significant, with profound implications for both overall health and well-being, as well as the likelihood of maintaining long-term weight loss.

Most people tend to focus on the aesthetic benefits of exercise or its role in enhancing athletic performance. However, an equally vital—though admittedly less sexy—benefit is that preserving muscle mass supports our ability to carry out everyday tasks that require strength and endurance. This, obviously, is especially important for older adults, as maintaining muscle mass helps counteract the age-related decline in physical strength, reducing the risks of frailty-related issues like falls and injuries.[328]

Moreover, as scientists continue to investigate the effects of physical activity and exercise, they are uncovering a growing list of health benefits that extend far beyond the physical aspect of muscle building. For example, the reduction in body fat percentage has been shown to correlate with improvements in a wide range of health factors.[329] These include reduction in blood pressure and proinflammatory markers, increased insulin sensitivity (meaning a lower risk of diabetes), lower cholesterol levels, a better ratio of saturated to unsaturated fats, favorable changes in blood lipids, lipoproteins, and hemostatic factors.[330] According to the CDC, the combined effects of these positive changes result in a demonstrable reduction in the risk of heart attack, stroke, and several types of cancer.[331]

Exercise also has a second, favorable impact more directly related to our primary focus here: it improves the prospects of *long-term success* in weight loss efforts. And it does so in a bona fide *Judo-esque* manner—by literally "muscling" our body to work for us rather than against us. How? You got it. By preserving and even increasing the fat-free body mass—the principal metabolically active component of total body mass—exercise partially blunts the reduction in metabolic activity that accompanies weight loss through dieting alone.[332]

Let's dive deeper to explore why this might very well be our "metabolic ace in the hole" for achieving sustainable, long-term weight-loss success!

A Bona fide *Judo-esque* move to Maintain Weight-loss

As previously explained, an important—yet often overlooked—impediment to weight loss efforts is the body's involuntary adaptation to conserve energy during caloric deprivation. This mechanism serves to minimize tissue loss and prevent the body from "withering away." Two mechanisms induce this reduction in energy expenditure. The first, and most significant—and the one already discussed—is the body's innate response to slow metabolic activity at the cellular level, thereby reducing maintenance energy expenditure (MEE). The second involves a smaller but still impactful drop in total energy expenditure stemming from a reduction in the energy expended during weight-bearing physical activities. Since most physical activities rely on muscle contractions to move the body or its parts, a person's body weight directly influences the amount of energy required for movement—the lighter the body, the less energy is expended during motion.[333,334]

The adaptation in MEE—which experimental research studies suggest can drop by as much as 20 percent—is, however, the dominant factor. Because MEE accounts for a whopping 60-70 percent of total daily energy expenditure for a typical sedentary adult, a 10-20 percent drop in MEE would constitute a significant drop, in absolute terms, in a person's total daily energy expenditure.[335,336,337] This becomes a serious, often unwelcome complication for a dieter striving to lose weight. (Remember: the physiological purpose of MEE suppression is to slow metabolic activity, thereby restraining the rate of tissue depletion— a survival mechanism for the body but the exact opposite of what a dieter aims to achieve.)

This raises a crucial question regarding long-term weight-loss maintenance: How long does this "MEE depression" last?

Until recently, the answer remained unclear—a lingering mystery. Budgetary constraints often limited the duration of experimental studies leaving scientists well-versed in the body's metabolic and hormonal adjustments *during weight-loss efforts* but with little understanding of their long-term effects. In 2009, however, a groundbreaking Australian study provided new insights.[338] The study monitored a group of 50 overweight men and women for several months following a weight-loss intervention. The findings revealed that these individuals remained in what could be described as a "biologically altered state" for a full year after their significant weight loss.

The study revealed that several hormones associated with hunger and metabolism—specifically leptin, ghrelin, and peptide YY—remained significantly altered compared to pre-dieting levels. (Leptin is a hormone that suppresses hunger and boosts metabolism, while ghrelin, often called the "hunger hormone," and peptide YY are both linked to hunger signals.) These persistent biological changes helped explain why participants (like so many dieters) experienced heightened hunger and reduced energy expenditure for many months after their weight-loss intervention. The researchers concluded that "… their still-plump bodies were acting as if they were starving and were working overtime to regain the pounds they lost."[339]

These results offer both diagnostic insight and a prescriptive lesson. They suggest that the high rate of weight-loss relapse is driven not only by voluntary behavior (such as the resumption of old habits) but also by significant physiological responses. And the prescriptive lesson: successful weight-loss maintenance is *not* automatic. It requires effective *and* sustainable strategies to counteract the body's compensatory mechanisms, which persist for months following weight loss.

While success in weight loss is all about creating and adhering to an *energy deficit*, weight-loss <u>maintenance</u> hinges on maintaining *energy balance* at a new, lower body size and a reduced energy expenditure level. The critical challenge—and the essence of the difficulty—lies in maintaining this balance *despite the reduction in energy expenditure,* which, as the research findings discussed above show, is both substantial and prolonged.

This points to practical tactics for long-term weight maintenance, which we'll explore next.

Don't Trade… Integrate

After weight-loss, "successful losers" may pursue one of three strategies to sustain energy balance at their reduced body size and lower energy expenditure: 1) Eat less—specifically, less than their pre-weight-loss intake—to offset the reduction in involuntary energy expenditure that accompanies weight loss; 2) Increase physical activity—beyond their pre-weight-loss level; or 3) Combine both approaches—reducing caloric intake while also increasing physical activity.[340]

Most people tend to focus primarily on the first strategy, seeking (hoping?) to maintain a permanent reduction in their caloric intake. The record, however, is pretty clear: most fail to sustain their weight loss long-term. The reason isn't hard to discern. In a world flooded with highly palatable, energy-dense, and easily accessible food, maintaining a permanent reduction in caloric intake requires extraordinary willpower to override the body's persistent psychophysiological urges to overeat and regain the weight.

Relying solely on increased physical activity (option 2) presents its own challenges. Thermodynamic principles underscore the difficulty: burning 300 calories—the equivalent of a single candy bar—may require a full hour of jogging. Extrapolating further, for a male dieter aiming to sustain a 10% or greater weight loss, this strategy might necessitate 40–80 minutes of moderate-to-vigorous physical activity daily. For many, this represents a prohibitive and unappealing commitment of time and effort, making it difficult to sustain over the long term.[341]

The third strategy—what I call the "Don't Trade... Integrate" approach—combines a moderate increase in physical activity with a *Judo-inspired* redesign of food intake. This approach emphasizes practical, palatable changes, such as reducing energy density to eat fewer calories without feeling deprived, while incorporating a manageable and sustainable exercise regimen. Many believe this balanced, integrated method offers the most promising and sustainable path forward.[342]

Incorporating regular exercise into your weight-loss maintenance plan helps ease the challenge of maintaining long-term energy balance by raising the threshold at which this balance must be maintained, reducing the need for drastic caloric cuts to sustain weight loss. To illustrate, consider a female dieter whose daily energy expenditure drops from 3,000 kcal to 2,000 kcal post weight-loss due to reduced body size and lower MEE. Maintaining her new weight without exercise would require a substantial 33% reduction in caloric intake—a significant burden to bear for months and months. As we've learned in Chapter 3, experimental studies consistently show that the greater the deprivation—which a 33% cut certainly qualifies as— the stronger the physiological "signal" sent to the brain's appetite-control center, urging us to: *"EAT, EAT, EAT."*

Incorporating exercise can help lessen the severity of—and even mitigate—the deprivation. For instance, adding a 500-kcal daily exercise routine—such as brisk walking for a few miles—raises her energy expenditure baseline from 2,000 to 2,500. But the benefits don't end there! Longer-term, exercise provides an additional "caloric bonus." Beyond the 500-kcal expended through *voluntary* physical activity (like brisk walking), exercise elevates the body's energy balance threshold by increasing MEE through the preservation and/or building of muscle mass. This *involuntary* increase in MEE can contribute an extra 100 kcal or more—a welcome addition that is far from insignificant.[343]

With this in mind, her daily caloric deficit would decrease to a more manageable 400-500 kcal—an amount that can be more easily achieved through moderate dietary adjustments rather than extreme caloric restriction. Indeed, by creatively redesigning her food intake using the strategies outlined in Chapter 4—such as reducing the average energy density of her meals—she could cut these 400-500 calories while remaining within *her satiating margin,* thus avoiding feelings of hunger. (Recall Dr. Brian Wansink's research at Cornell, which suggests that each person has a range of meal sizes—*a satiated or gratified margin*—within which they feel content and satiated after a meal.[344])

The prize? No hunger pain, no weight gain!

The evidence supporting the efficacy of the "Don't Trade... Integrate" strategy is robust and continues to grow. In one prototypical study, researcher compared the self-reported activity levels of three groups of women: obese women who regained weight after successful weight loss (labelled as "relapsers"), formerly obese women who maintained their weight loss ("maintainers"), and normal-weight women who maintained their weight (the controls).[345]

The findings were striking: 90% of *maintainers* and 82% of *controls* reported engaging in regular physical activity—defined as at least three sessions per week of 30 minutes or more. In contrast, only 34% of *relapsers* reported the same. These results underscore the critical role of consistent physical activity in maintaining weight—both for individuals of normal weight and for those who have lost a significant amount of weight.

But perhaps the strongest (and most widely cited) evidence comes from the National Weight Control Registry, the largest U.S. study of successful weight-loss maintainers:

> Almost 100 percent of them use a combination of diet and exercise to lose weight, and about 95 percent use a combination of diet and exercise to maintain their loss.... How much exercise? Far more than the recommended minimum. On average they expend 2,800 kcal (12 MJ) a week through physical activity, the equivalent of walking four miles a day every day, although most use a mixture of different activities, including walking, aerobic dancing, tennis, cycling, running and lifting weights.[346]

A Gift that Keeps on Giving

Exercise has one more thing going for it: like food, it can be rewarding—even addictive. But unlike the obesifying rewards of food, it is a healthy kind of addiction!

> A substantial body of science tells us that exercise engages the same neural regions as other mood-enhancing rewards and produces similar chemical responses. Just as a smoker thinks he needs a cigarette; someone who exercises regularly comes to depend on the positive effects it produces.
>
> Exercise can also reinforce an altered self-image. You begin to identify yourself as a healthy, athletic person, someone capable of making positive choices, and that in turn gives you an incentive to maintain control. New habits begin to substitute for old ones, making it easier to stay faithful to your eating plan.[347]

As we exercise more and more, our skills naturally improve, and our physiological capacity expands—with enhancements such as increased lung capacity, stronger heart function, and greater muscle endurance.[348] As the physiological capacity for physical exertion grows, we can exercise longer and harder, which leads to further improvements. It is the quintessential *virtuous* cycle: an initial change—such as improved strength, flexibility, stamina—builds upon itself, creating a snowball effect that amplifies the benefits (Figure 6.3).

The result? The more we exercise, the better and better we feel about ourselves and about exercising, which motivates us to exercise even more. It's a powerful, positive feedback loop that transforms exercise from a simple choice into a rewarding, ongoing journey.

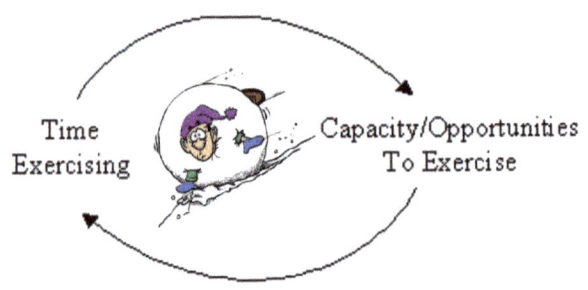

Figure 6.3
The virtuous cycle of exercising acts as a snowball accumulating mass as it rolls downhill

Chapter 7

Beyond Physiology: The Challenges of Self-Regulation

Mental *O goshi*

While Judo's techniques were originally conceived as martial arts fighting skills, its underlying tenets—training the body and cultivating the mind to perform at "maximum efficiency"— are, as discussed in Chapter 2, *universal principles* that apply to a wide spectrum of human behavior... beyond combat. Dr. Jigoro Kano, the father of Judo, consistently emphasized in his writings and teachings that the essence of its *Seiryoku-Zenyo* principle—making the most efficient use of mental and physical energy to achieve one's goals—has broad relevance to everyday life. He fervently urged his disciples to apply Judo's precepts well beyond the *dojo*, integrating them into their daily lives.

In Chapters 4 through 6, we focused on applying Judo's principles to work with, rather than against, the body's *physical* processes—specifically, those governing energy-in (eating) and energy-out (exercise). In this chapter, we extend these principles to the *cognitive* domain, addressing the challenges of self-control. Just as in the physical realm, the *Seiryoku Zenyo* principle of maximum efficiency is equally applicable—and just as effective. Our ability to self-regulate is essential for successful weight-loss maintenance, and because—as we will fully explain— the human capacity to self-regulate is a limited resource, it needs to be efficiently managed and must not be squandered.

The Challenges of Self-Control

When individuals reduce food intake while dieting, they do so not because their physiology signals it, but for personal reasons that often conflict with their natural physiological drives. These reasons are cognitive and deliberate, not physiological and automatic.[349] Indeed, humans are the only species on the planet in which hungry individuals will voluntarily refuse to consume readily available, appealing food in pursuit of an aesthetic or health goal.[350,351]

However, this is not always an easy thing to pull off.

> In principle, performing almost any behavior should require more exertion than not performing it. Eating a piece of pie, for example, requires various muscular movements of arm, fingers, and jaw. Yet most dieters can attest that refraining from such behaviors can seem more difficult and draining than performing them.
> In such cases, refraining from the desired behavior involves more than mere passive inaction: Refraining from behaving requires an act of self-control by which the self alters its own behavioral patterns so as to prevent or inhibit its dominant response. A hungry person would normally respond to desirable food by eating it, and so a dieter requires some internal process to prevent that response.
> That internal process may require a form of exertion that seems more difficult and strenuous than eating.[352]

In dieting, as with many forms of self-regulation, there is an inner conflict pulling us in opposite directions (Figure 7.1). This conflict pits the cognitive against the physiological—between the desire to stick to a strict diet and the urge to "… gobble down that doughnut someone has placed on the table in front of you."[353]

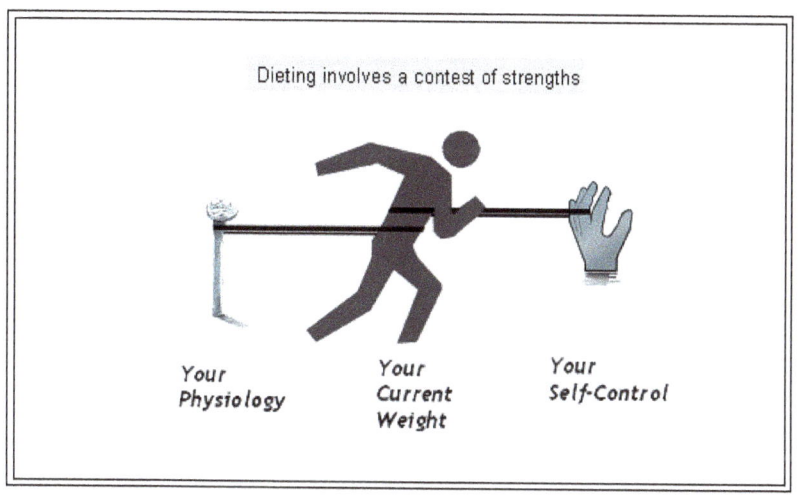

Figure 7.1: Conflict between the cognitive and physiologic

As an act of self-control, dieting to lose weight or maintain weight loss is much like resisting temptations, persevering through tiring tasks, breaking bad habits, and the like—a process in which the self exerts control over itself.[354] We engage in self-regulation whenever we inhibit immediate desires or gratification, or refrain from acting on strong but undesirable impulses.[355]

This capacity to self-regulate, as in all above examples and countless more, is truly among the most extraordinary and impressive of human functions. "It has provided us with an adaptive edge that enabled our ancestors to survive and even flourish when changing conditions led other species to extinction."[356] On a personal level, our ability (or lack thereof) to regulate ourselves shapes our sense of self and is a key determinant of success (or failure) across many spheres of life, including family, school, business, and health.[357,358,359]

In recent years, there has been growing recognition of the role self-regulation plays in health and weight management. Below, I provide a brief overview of the influential *self-control strength model,* and explain its important implications for personal health regulation.

The Self-Control Strength Model

Roy F. Baumeister, Dianne Tice, Mark Muraven (all of Case Western Reserve University), along with Todd Heatherton (of Harvard), are credited with formulating the *strength model of human self-regulation*.[360,361] The model helps explain self-control performance, not only in static terms, such as differences among individuals or by type of task, but also dynamically—e.g., the persistence and duration of the self-control effort over time. Thanks to their work, we now have a better understanding of the self-regulatory process—both its theoretical importance and practical utility—and its indispensable role in the self-regulation of personal health.

The model has three core principles:

- The act of self-regulation is an effortful process that requires strength to override impulses and resist temptations.[362]
- The human capacity for self-regulation operates like a muscle—it is a limited resource that is partially depleted during self-control efforts. Acts of self-control not only require the use of strength, but also reduce the amount of strength available for subsequent self-control efforts. Like muscular strength, self-control strength is replenished with rest after exertion.[363]
- Self-control performance depends on both an individual's level of self-control strength—the availability of the resource—and their motivation to exert self-control—its mobilization.[364] In other words, motivation and available self-control strength jointly determine the extent of self-control exerted.[365]

Self-control strength may thus be conceptualized as a reservoir or stock that is depleted and replenished over time, with self-control exertion depleting it and rest restoring it. This stock-and-flow structure (see Figure 7.2 below) mirrors the plumbing analogy from Chapter 5, which we used to illustrate the dynamics—the rise and fall—of energy reserves in the human body. This is not merely a coincidence; it exemplifies a key systems-thinking insight: systems across diverse domains—whether biological, engineering, or social—*share common structural patterns.*

It is an empowering insight that allows us to repurpose and extend our understanding, knowledge and skill from one familiar problem domain—such as managing the reservoir of water in a tub or energy/fat in the human body—to other, perhaps less transparent, systems like self-control. This is precisely what we will explore here.

This is a skill that can serve us well. These stock-and-flow structures (their academic term) are ubiquitous in our lives, extending beyond weight regulation, self-control… and bathtubs. Consider your car's gas tank, or, if you drive an electric vehicle (EV), your battery's charge. These dual automotive examples are particularly enlightening, as they both involve identical stock-and-flow systems—a fuel stock that you replenish at a gas or charging station and deplete when driving. However, while their structures are similar, their complexities are anything but. Managing an EV's stock, for example, presents additional challenges. Just ask any EV owner about "range anxiety"—the fear of running out of battery power before reaching a charging station. This reflects the unique challenge EV owners face in managing their vehicle's stock-and-flow fueling system. Not only is the full-charge range of most EVs relatively limited (typically between 200 and 500 miles), but it also fluctuates significantly based on driving habits and weather conditions (cold weather can reduce an EV's range by as much as 30%). As we'll see shortly, there are intriguing parallels between these challenges and those of self-control, despite the obvious contrast between the two domains.

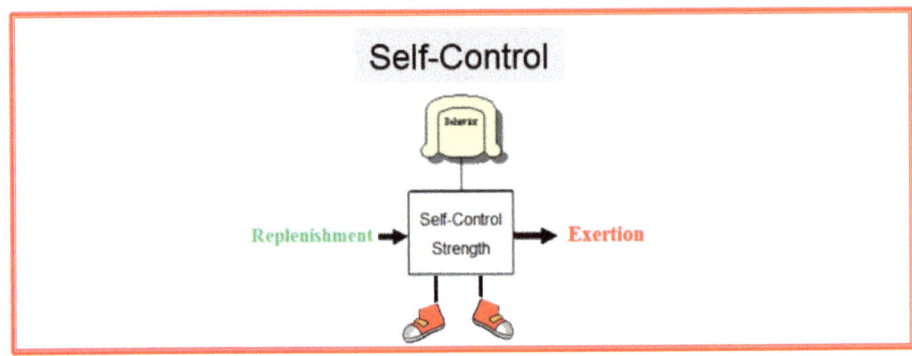
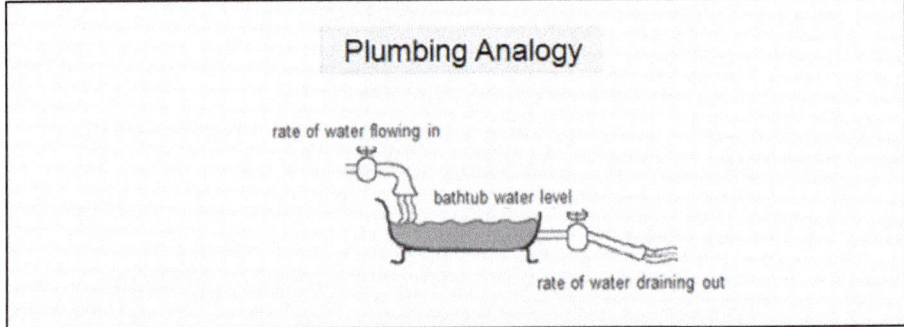
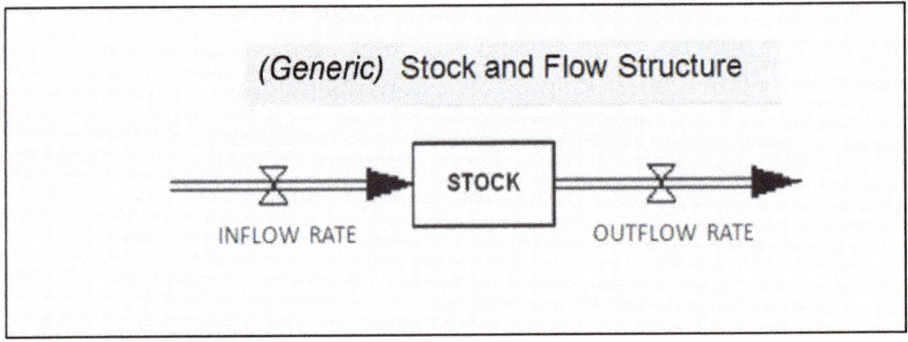

Figure 7.2: Self-control follows a stock-and-flow structure: it depletes with exertion and replenishes with rest

When managing stock-and-flow systems—whether it's fuel in a car or self-control energy—a fundamental question we, as the protagonists, must address is how best to manage a limited resource to achieve a desired goal (e.g., reaching a distant destination). In the case of managing a gas tank—still the most common car type—this means understanding that driving speed significantly impacts fuel consumption. The faster you drive, the higher the rate of fuel consumption, the lower the miles per gallon, and, consequently, the fewer miles you can travel on a full tank. Analogously, in weight-loss, we'll see that aggressive ("high velocity") strategies—say aiming to lose fifteen pounds in a week—deplete our self-control capacity at a higher (and possibly unsustainable) rate than a slower approach, like aiming to lose the same amount over a month (half a pound a day). Just like a car's fuel tank, our "tank" of self-control strength is not limitless, so it must be managed wisely *to go the distance.*

No matter the system—mechanical, plumbing, or biological—stock-and-flow systems all function in fundamentally the same way, following the rules of accumulation and depletion, though there may be important nuances in their complexity. Given the ubiquity of such systems in our lives—and their crucial role in regulating our bodies and well-being—it's essential that we: (1) recognize them, and (2) master the skills needed to regulate their replenishment and depletion rates.

Regulation of Energy Reservoirs: Physical and Psychological

For *any* stock or reservoir, the fundamental laws of conservation, accumulation and depletion are straightforward: the relative rates of flow into and out of the stock govern how the quantity (or level) of the stock changes over time. For example, if the outflow exceeds the inflow, the stock level will gradually decrease and, given enough time, it may fully deplete. In many stock-and-flow systems, complete depletion can be problematic—and sometimes even catastrophic. This is true, for example, when driving a vehicle on a route with few refueling stations. It also applies to self-control.

If, and how fast, depletion of a stock occurs will depend on the initial size of the stock and the magnitude of the imbalance between inflow and outflow. Hence, the key to regulating a stock's level and avoiding catastrophic depletion is to manage the relative magnitudes of the inflow and outflows rates. This principle applies to mechanical systems, like a car, as well as human systems, both physical and psychological.

Let's first consider a *physical* human activity—such as muscular exertion—since it's easier to visualize. In this case, the body has two primary energy stores (or "tanks")—one for fat and the other for glycogen (the form in which carbohydrates are stored). Both tanks function similarly, though they differ in size and serve distinct purposes. On the former, the difference in size between our fat and glycogen stores is enormous—our fat stores are nearly fifty times larger.[366] This is no evolutionary accident. Fat contains twice the energy per unit weight of carbohydrates—nine kilocalories per gram of fat compared to four kilocalories per gram of carbohydrate—making fat a highly efficient and compact energy storage solution. This enables us to carry a substantial energy reserve without being slowed down, which is a significant advantage when an individual (or animal) must be highly motile to survive.[367]

Besides differences in "tank" size, the two fuels serve different functions. Carbohydrate-based fuel provides faster energy transfer and can be used anaerobically—meaning, it can be metabolized to produce energy without the simultaneous use of oxygen. This makes it the ideal fuel to use for activities that need immediate bursts of energy—i.e., whenever we perform at a rate that exceeds the capacity of the heart and lungs to supply oxygen to the muscles—such as sprinting to catch a bus, win a squash game, or escape a charging rhino.

Yet, the filling and draining of the two tanks function in the same way. Energy in the tank—whether fat or glycogen—is depleted when we exert muscular energy, and replenished by ingesting food energy (fats and carbohydrates). (Note: Besides carbohydrate and fat, the human diet provides a third macronutrient: protein. The primary task of proteins is to provide the major building blocks for the synthesis of body tissue.[368])

The balance between inflow and outflow rates—nutritional energy replenishment versus muscular exertion—along with the size of the body's energy stores, which depend on an individual's body composition and physical conditioning, determines whether a particular activity will deplete energy reserves and constrain physical performance. For someone living a sedentary lifestyle, the muscular exertion involved in daily activities such as walking, cooking, working at the office, shopping, etc. are typically modest. In these cases, the drain on energy reserves—mostly from the body's fat stores—is slow enough that it is adequately compensated for by daily food intake, resulting in no noticeable decline in performance.

However, this state of relative stability can shift dramatically during *intense* physical activity. As noted earlier, when a person exercises at high intensity, the muscles must tap into the body's limited glycogen reserves to obtain the glucose needed to fuel the work. The higher the intensity of physical activity, the faster the glycogen drain rate. Since the human body's glycogen reserves are relatively small—only a few hundred grams, amounting to roughly 2,500 kcal—they can sustain only one to two hours of intense exertion before being exhausted.[369] Once depleted, muscle fatigue sets in, diminishing our capacity to continue exercising.

Now, let's consider the *psychological* case.

Just as humans are able to sustain low-intensity physical exertion throughout daily activities, we also know from personal experience that we're capable of maintaining modest levels of self-control day in and day out. This suggests that the amount of self-control required for daily social functioning—stopping at a stop sign, standing in line when in a hurry, holding our tempers, and so forth—is modest enough that normal periods of rest can compensate for the slow depletion rate. Indeed, many scholars have argued that the human capacity to inhibit antisocial impulses—and being able to do it all day long—has been a key facilitator, even a necessary condition, of civilized life.[370,371]

But what about situations where we need to—or choose to—exert *more-than-modest* levels of self-control, such as resisting the urge to eat even when persistently hungry? Not eating under such circumstances clearly demands far more self-control than resisting the temptation to speed on the highway. And having to sustain the effort over an extended period raises an important question: what happens when we exert more-than-modest levels of self-control to resist stronger, more persistent impulses? Can normal periods of rest compensate for the increased and sustained depletion of self-regulation, or is the human capacity for self-regulation—much like our glycogen stores—a limited resource that depletes relatively quickly under intense exertion?

It is an important question, one that demanded an empirical resolution. Researchers in self-control needed to assess whether the human capacity (stock) for self-control is sufficient enough to sustain periods of intense and prolonged exertion without significant deterioration.

Over the past two decades, a wide range of studies have been conducted to assess self-regulatory depletion in humans. These include experiments in controlled laboratory settings as well as analyses of autobiographical accounts detailing individuals' self-regulation experiences—both successes and failures.[372]

Many of these studies were carried out by Professor Baumeister's research group at Case Western Reserve University.[373] A primary focus of their laboratory experiments was to assess how people perform when engaged in a series of self-regulatory tasks. In a typical experiment, participants were asked to exert self-control during an initial task, and their performance was then measured on a subsequent, often different, task.[374]

The experiments encompassed a variety of challenges, including traditional forms of self-control, such as delaying gratification or resisting temptations like eating, smoking, or drinking alcohol. They also involved tasks requiring persistence in frustrating mental exercises, such as solving difficult anagrams, and endurance in the face of physical discomfort, such as athletic or manual-labor tasks that demanded continued effort despite fatigue.[375]

The results across these studies were remarkably consistent and led to a clear conclusion: The capacity for self-regulation, much like muscular strength, is a limited resource subject to temporary depletion.[376] As individuals exert self-control, their ability to sustain it gradually diminishes.[377] Baumeister and colleagues put it succinctly: "To use it is to lose it, at least temporarily."[378] The bit of good news, however, is that the degradation in self-control strength is not permanent. With adequate rest—and, in particular, sleep—people typically regain their lost capacity for self-regulation.

The researchers expected, and found, individual differences in both innate capacity for self-regulation and the motivation to mobilize one's reserves. As we observe in daily life, some people are much better than others at holding their tempers, sticking to their diets, stopping after a couple of drinks, saving money, persevering at work, and so on.[379] The experiments not only confirmed these impressions but also empirically demonstrated that the differences in individuals' degrees of self-regulation can be substantial. In other words, when it comes to self-control strength, some people have a much larger stock than others.[380,381]

The researchers also found that *incentives* significantly influenced self-control performance. When participants were offered stronger incentives, they exerted more self-control and consequently performed better on tasks requiring it. Tasks with inherently more appealing outcomes or a higher likelihood of success also increased motivation, leading to better self-control performance—provided the exertion did not deplete their self-control reserves.[382]

Interestingly, experimental results also revealed that—much like muscular exertion—self-regulation in one area diminished the ability to self-regulate in another.[383] This suggests that different self-regulatory tasks draw on the same reservoir. In other words, a single capacity appears to underlie the full range of self-regulatory functions, and "any and all attempts at self-control require the use of this resource."[384]

Since the same resource is used for many (or conceivably all) acts of self-control, we would hope that it's a large resource. Apparently, it is not. The findings indicate that, for most people, this resource is rather limited. In many of these experiments, acts of self-regulation were relatively brief, yet performance was significantly degraded on subsequent tasks.[385]

An important and obvious implication of these results is that our capacity for self-regulation needs to be managed like any other *limited* resource—and must not be squandered.[386] Since we have little control over the size of our "tank" (or stock)—at least in the short term—our success or failure in self-control, particularly in taxing endeavors, will largely depend on how we manage the capacity we have—a choice we *do* control.

So, how effective are dieters at managing their limited capacity for self-regulation? On this, the record is clear: not particularly well—with plenty of clues as to why.

Irrational Exuberance… and its Perils

While most dieters are undoubtedly aware that they would have a better chance of success with reasonable weight-loss goals—whether in terms of the ultimate weight target, the pace to achieve it, or both—setting more realistic goals often doesn't align most dieters' personal agendas. Nor are they encouraged to. The diet industry thrives for two reasons: big promises and repeat customers. The big promises attract the customers in the first place, and the magnitude of the promises virtually guarantees that they cannot be fulfilled. It makes for a very attractive business model![387]

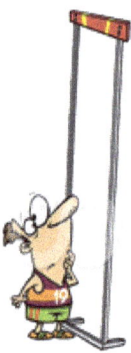

Research suggests that most dieters pay a hefty price for their irrational exuberance. The unrealistic goals they set not only make success virtually unattainable but, even worse, often contribute to relapse.

But why?

The greater the weight-loss goal, the greater the caloric deficit must be. The greater the caloric deficit, the more acute the hunger and the greater the self-control needed to override the deprivation and sustain the diet—in other words, the greater the depletion rate of the dieter's self-control capacity (or stock). That much is obvious. What may be less apparent, however, is how much harder it becomes and how quickly the hardship escalates.

Dieters can seriously underestimate the escalation in hardship because, as psychologists have found, most people intuitively view causality in *linear* terms, expecting effect to be proportional to cause. That is to say, we to tend to think that if A causes B, then doubling A will produce twice as much B. In dieting terms, this leads people to believe that losing 2 pounds a week will require only twice the effort of losing 1 pound a week.

But the effort needed to accomplish a task often increases *exponentially*, not linearly, as the difficulty of the task increases. In other words, if achieving A requires expending B, doubling the target to 2 A's will often more than double the cost—requiring say the expenditure of 4 B's (not just 2). This principle is not unique to dieting, it applies to many tasks, both cognitive and physical.

Consider, for instance, walking, which for most people is the primary form of physical activity in a relatively sedentary lifestyle. The "Escalating Energy Expenditure" plot in Figure 7.3, portrays how energy expenditure escalates as walking speed increases, from 1 to 10 km per hour (0.62 to 6.2 mph). It shows that as speed increases, energy expenditure rises, but not in a linear fashion. It rises exponentially. (Interestingly, the plot of driving speed versus fuel consumption has a very similar pattern!)

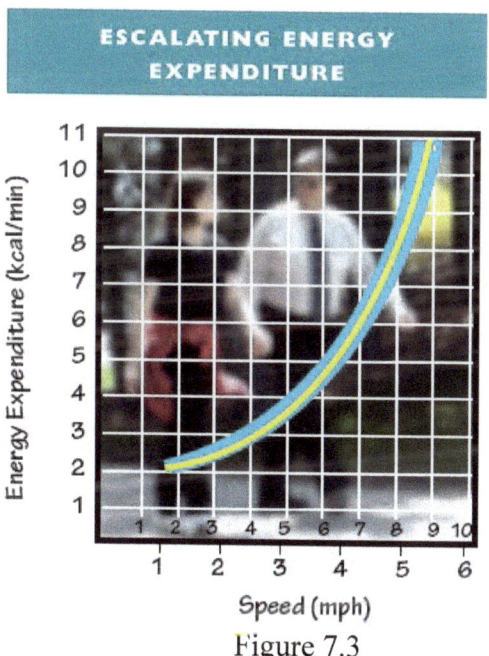

Figure 7.3

Energy expended while walking, as a function of speed

At low walking speeds—around the one- to two-mph pace typical of daily activities—the exertion of muscular energy, which reflects the outflow rate of the body's energy stock, is modest enough that the drain on energy reserves can be adequately compensated for by daily rest and moderate food intake (the inflow rate of energy into the body). In other words, this level of exertion is *sustainable*, meaning we could maintain this level of physical activity for extended periods without depleting our muscular energy stock.

In fact, we can sustain it almost indefinitely, as evidenced by Deborah De Williams. On Friday, October 15, 2004, De Williams returned to her hometown of Melbourne after setting a world record as the first woman to walk around Australia—traveling clockwise along Australia's National Highway 1 (http://www.walkaroundoz.org.au/). She completed the 9,715-mile walk in 343 days, earning a second world record for the "longest walk in the shortest time." Deborah De Williams had walked close to 30 miles per day, at a speed of two miles per hour—which translates to 15 hours of walking each day, every day, for almost an entire year. This is an indubitable manifestation of sustained energy stock, if there ever was one.

As the walking speed versus energy-expenditure plot in Figure 7.3 illustrates, walking faster can quickly increase the rate of energy expenditure. Running would escalate it further still. Once our rate of energy expenditure exceeds our ability to replenish our reserves, they begin to deplete over time. How quickly? Consider what it takes to run a marathon. The human energy "stock" (even for the best stocked individuals) is barely large enough to sustain a 26-mile marathon run—quite a bit less than De Williams' 9,715 miles. And those resilient enough to endure that challenge will most certainly arrive with empty tanks.

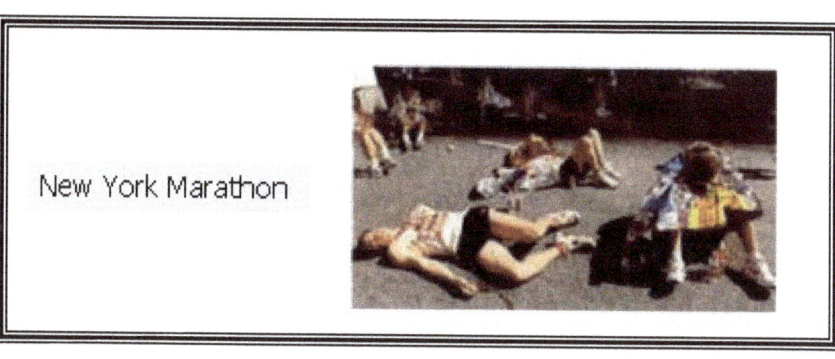
New York Marathon

Much like walking or running, the self-regulatory effort in weight loss escalates not linearly, but exponentially, as the difficulty of the goal increases. Our body's weight *set point*— the specific weight range that each individual's body naturally tries to maintain through hormonal and metabolic mechanisms—seems to have a certain give to it, so that a person can stay a bit below it with relatively little effort. Larger weight losses, on the other hand, are difficult to tolerate.

Fat-cell theory (as discussed in Chapter 3) provides one possible mechanism for this physiological nonlinearity. As the enlarged fat cells of an overweight dieter—which would have expanded in size during weight gain to accommodate excess energy storage—shrink back to their normal size (or slightly below it) with *modest* weight loss, the gentle (nonchalant) physiological signals to overeat and regain the weight are often easy to override. But if the weight-loss effort persists and the fat cells deplete to levels much below normal, the "volume" of the physiological message to the brain's appetite-control center to "EAT," amplifies, eventually becoming a scream.

Experimental studies show just how "deafening" the message can become. In acute-dieting experiments, seriously overweight individuals who lost large amounts of weight developed a psychiatric syndrome called semi-starvation neurosis—a condition previously observed in individuals of normal weight who had been starved. These distressed subjects continuously fantasized about food or about breaking their diet; they dreamed of food and became anxious and depressed, and some even had thoughts of suicide.[388]

The bottom line: Higher goals deplete the energy stock faster than it can be replenished, leading to failure—much like a marathoner who sprints early, only to run out of energy later. The harder we push, the harder the body pushes back. The greater the weight loss, the stronger the sensation of hunger and the drive to eat and, hence, the greater the exertion of self-control and the higher the risk of self-control depletion.[389] Because successful weight-loss is not just about how much we lose initially, but also about sustaining the loss long-term—an effortful self-regulatory process—self-control stock depletion inevitably leads to relapse.

Adding insult to injury, failure rarely prompts genuine self-reflection or course correction. In situations like dieting, where our self-esteem is on the line, we are naturally biased to interpret failure in a way that preserves our positive self-image—for instance, blaming the specific diet we used rather than our unrealistic expectations. And resolving to try anew to attain our lofty goals, but this time with whatever the latest diet trend happens to be. The all-too-familiar result: getting trapped in a recurring cycle of weight loss and regain—what's colloquially known as "*Yo-Yo* dieting."

The *Yo-Yo* Trap

Most people erroneously assume that there is no serious downside to setting an unrealistic weight loss goal. That shooting for one's "dream" body weight, no matter how unreasonable, will at worst land us at whatever achievable level we would have attained anyways. This is the scenario depicted in Figure 7.4, showing a dieter falling short of her dream goal level, but ending up at the level she assumes she would have attained anyways had she started her diet aiming for that more modest (and achievable) goal. A level she also expects she can and will sustain (self-control wise). So, no harm done, right? Wrong.

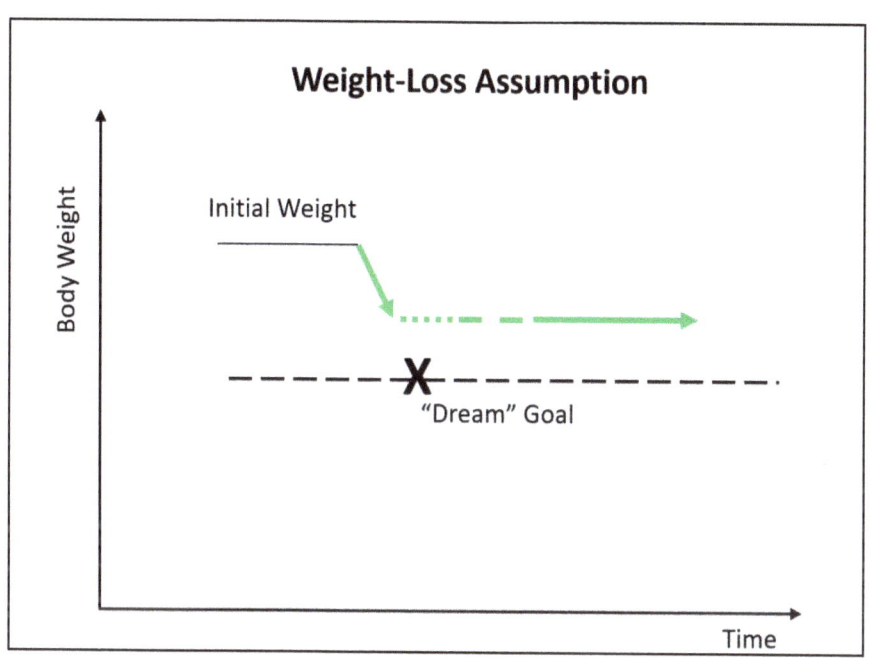

Figure 7.4
Weight-loss assumption

In reality, setting an unrealistic goal can take an unsuspecting dieter on a *wilder* ride… and ultimately leading to relapse (Figure 7.5a). In the all-too-familiar pattern, dieters seeking lofty weight-loss goals may be able to initially slash off large amounts of weight by eating very little or even starving themselves, but then run out of regulatory gas. The inevitable result: after a period of short-lived success, they regain the weight back—often with "interest."[390] For these dieters—and they are, by far, the majority—the end result leaves them worse off than if they had started with and maintained a more modest weight-loss goal—the sustainable path depicted in Figure 7.5b.

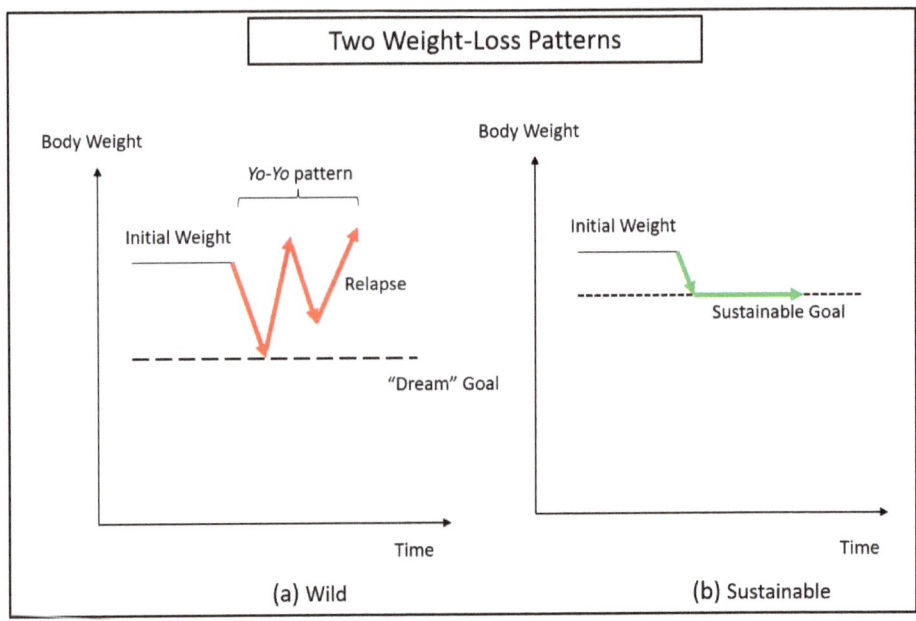

Figure 7.5
"Wild" versus Sustainable paths

Whether we're managing body weight, personal finances, or gasoline consumption, the goal we set not only defines the *endpoint* of an endeavor, but also shapes the *path* to achieving it. Therefore, establishing a *different* goal can *create* an entirely different trajectory and, quite possibly, a very different outcome. (Academics refer to situations where the final outcome of an endeavor depends on the path we choose as "path dependence.") It is an important lesson to heed to effectively manage many of our affairs—professional and personal—including managing personal health.

With all this mind, let's recap.

When pondering a diet, remember: the greater the weight-loss goal, the greater the caloric deficit will be. The greater the caloric deficit, the more acute the dieter's hunger and the greater the self-control energy needed to override the deprivation and sustain the diet—that is, the greater the drain on the dieter's reservoir of self-control capacity. And as demonstrated experimentally by Professor Baumeister's group, because the capacity for self-regulation is a limited resource, intense exertion leads to temporary depletion.[391]

With a depleted self-control stock, a dieter's capacity to adhere to her self-imposed caloric restriction erodes. As adherence to the diet progressively wanes, body weight invariably rebounds. Regaining the pounds, in turn, often saps the dieter's motivation, undermines belief in self-efficacy, and ultimately may drive dieters to give up, further accelerating the relapse.

Given the tremendous cultural pressure to be thin, this, however, seldom dissuades people from trying again. Weeks or months later—with rest and the replenishment of the self-control stock—the "irrationally exuberant" dieter may be back on the starting line for yet another trip on the weight-loss roller-coaster.

But wiser? Hardly ever.

In one revealing study, a group of overweight women—all repeat dieters—participating in a weight-loss program were asked to identify their desired weights before starting their new effort. Their target weights amounted to a whopping 32 percent reduction from their initial weight. This goal wasn't just ambitious in theoretical terms—far exceeding the five to ten percent reduction commonly recommended by experts and seen in the most successful weight-loss studies— but also unrealistic given the women's *own* past performance. On average, it was three times greater than what they had actually lost in previous attempts, suggesting that personal experience had done little to temper their "unhindered gusto."

These women are *no* outliers!

Research consistently finds that people tend to be overly optimistic when predicting outcomes, no matter their challenge.[392] When they fail to meet these inflated expectations, they often display remarkable skill in concocting convincing explanations—whether by blaming the shortcomings of the particular diet or other factors—to justify clinging to their unrealistic beliefs.[393] One of the most pernicious patterns in dieting is to "[blame] the failure on not having had enough willpower, with a simultaneous commitment to starting the diet again, but this time promising to try harder."[394]

All too often, this is reinforced by external agents:

First and foremost, testimonials provided by others who have allegedly succeeded using the same diet imply that the fault in one's own case must lie in oneself rather than in the diet... [Second,] the promoters of the diet in question have a vested interest in blaming the dieter rather than the diet. If the dieter consults the diet promoter—be it her doctor, her friend, the clinic where the diet program was obtained—she is likely to be told that she is at fault, in what amounts to classic instance of blaming the victim. The victim, who has supposedly failed to make the full effort required for success, has before her the opportunity to redeem herself by trying harder next time. Failure is due to an attributionally unstable characteristic [effort] and is therefore correctable.[395]

No matter the rationalization, the jeopardy people face when stubbornly clinging to unrealistic expectations—rather than honestly reflecting on and questioning the efficacy of their assumptions and strategies—is becoming trapped in repeating cycles of weight loss and regain.[396] When this extends over many years, the cyclic weight pattern often gets superimposed upon a longer-term upward drift in body weight. (As noted in Chapter 6, people tend to gain weight as they age because they burn fewer calories due to changes in body composition—such as loss of muscle mass—and a decrease in physical activity.) Figure 7.6 presents one of the precious few studies that tracked variations in body weight patterns over extended periods in free-living subjects. It shows the average weights of 31 women over a 25-year period. Over that time, this group of women—whose average age was 40—dieted an average of five times.[397] Notice how, as the women's weights cycled between weight loss and regain, their weights also steadily increased over time.

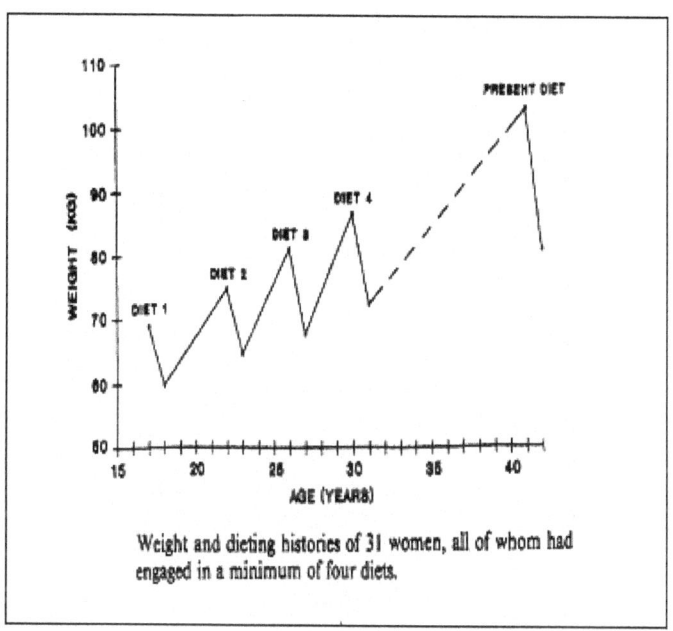

Figure 7.6
Weight-cycling superimposed over upward drift in body weight

There are at least two mechanisms through which yo-yo dieting itself contributes to such an upward drift in weight. First, when dieters fall short in their futile efforts, famished and disheartened, they often indulge in overeating binges.[398,399] The urge to overeat, especially after a period of acute dieting, is often driven by the psychological pressures and frustrations that build-up during food deprivation.[400,401] Second, some studies have found that repeated cycles of weight loss and regain are associated with increased metabolic efficiency, making subsequent dieting more difficult and predisposing individuals to weight gain.[402]

Although weight cycling is undoubtedly a source of frustration for many dieters, it is important to point out that the risks associated with repeated cycles of weight loss and regain go far beyond mere disappointment. A substantial body of epidemiologic research shows that repeated cycles of weight loss and regain increase the risks of chronic diseases—particularly coronary heart disease—and even premature death, independent of obesity itself.[403,404]

Weight cycling has also been found to have serious long-term "psychic costs," including loss of self-esteem, depressive mood states, and overall life dissatisfaction.[405,406] Repeated failures to attain expected weight-loss targets can gradually erode *self-efficacy*—that all important feeling of confidence to overcome obstacles and achieve desired outcomes.[407,408,409,410]

In summary, like any other limited and exhaustible resource, self-regulatory capacity needs to be managed and must not be squandered. Unfortunately, dieters rarely do this, nor are they encouraged to. The unrealistic goals that people set escalate self-regulatory exertion, leading to depletion and ultimately relapse.

Thankfully, however, things may be changing.

The Fog is Lifting: Goals Matter, and less May be More

A growing understanding of the biological factors that regulate body weight, along with the cognitive strain of maintaining large weight losses, is prompting a redefinition of what constitutes "success" in weight-loss programs. Slowly but surely, moderation is becoming the guiding principle of weight-loss efforts. A major catalyst for this shift is the growing evidence that moderate weight losses of just 10–15 percent of initial weight—even among substantially overweight individuals—are associated with significant improvements in nearly all parameters of health. These include blood pressure, heart morphology and functioning, lipid profile, glucose tolerance (especially among diabetics), sleep quality, and respiratory function. As a result, many federal agencies and health organizations are now advocating for more realistic weight-loss goals, rather than the pursuit of an "ideal" weight.

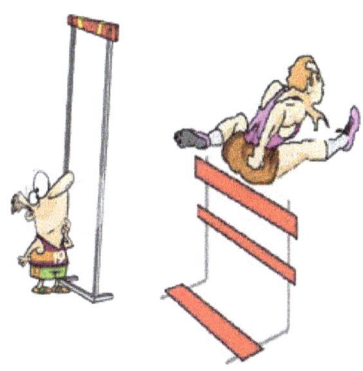

Moderating our weight-loss goals—whether for the ultimate target weight, the pace to achieve it, or both—reduces self-control exertion and improves the prospects of reaching our goal on a "tank-full" of self-control energy. It is the *judo-esque* course to work with your body, not against it. In this case, making the most efficient use of one's mental and self-control energy in the pursuit of one's weight-loss goals. On my "score sheet," this checks the second box of the *Seiryoku-Zenyo* principle I'm espousing: "making the most efficient use of one's physical (#1) and *mental energy* (#2) in pursuing one's goals." (In chapters 4 through 6, we checked box #1, covering judo-esque strategies pertaining to the *physical*—such as what and how we eat and how to "muscle" our body to work for us rather than against us.)

In practice, figuring out what works best for each individual—what weight-loss target to set, at what velocity and with what meal size and composition—will be a highly personal journey requiring experimentation and honest self-reflection. Unlike running out of gas when driving, when it comes to self-control, there isn't going to be an obvious "fuel gauge" or red flashing light to signal depletion. Hence, you'll need to watch for subtle, easily overlooked signs that you're "running on fumes."

Baumeister offers some hints on what to keep an eye on:

Do things seem to bother you more than they should? Has the volume somehow been turned up on your life so that things are felt more strongly than usual? Is it suddenly hard to make up your mind about even simple things? Are you more than usually reluctant to make a decision or exert yourself mentally or physically? If you notice such feelings, then reflect on the last few hours [meals?] and see if it seems likely that you have depleted your willpower.[411]

Finally, remember that self-control performance depends not only on self-control strength—how much an individual has in the tank—but also on the motivation to exert self-control. Adopting reasonable goals is beneficial on both fronts: it helps prevent dieters from running out of regulatory "gas" in the short term as well as guard against sapping their motivation and self-efficacy, both of which are essential for maintaining weight loss over the long term.

In Chapter 6, I discussed the potential benefits of harnessing the power of reinforcing feedback in exercising. That same dynamic applies here. Achieving or exceeding reasonable goals provides rewards instead of disappointments. Research studies have shown that this can create a virtuous, self-reinforcing cycle (see Figure 7.7). In one study, participants with higher levels of self-efficacy (assessed before a weight-loss intervention) were more successful in achieving their realistic weight-loss targets. In turn, reaching those targets strengthened their confidence and belief in their abilities, leading to better long-term outcomes in maintaining weight loss.[412]

Simply put: success begets success. Self-efficacy enhances weight-loss efforts, and successful weight loss bolsters self-efficacy. With each cycle around this positive feedback loop, the effect grows stronger as the process feeds on itself—undoubtedly a boon in the lifelong project to maintain a healthy weight in today's obesogenic environment.

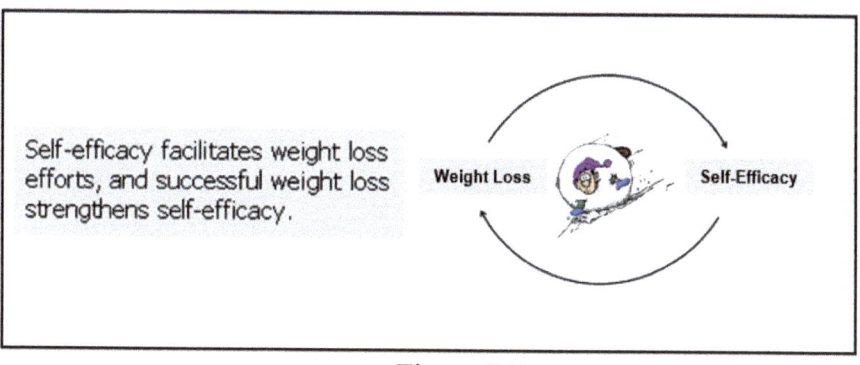

Figure 7.7
Success begets more success

Part III

Closing Argument: *Don't Delay*

Having discussed the tactics for managing weight gain and loss, we conclude in *Part III* (Chapter 8) by emphasizing that *when* we act is just as important as *how* we act.

As William Shakespeare, the sage of timeless wisdom, reminds us:

Make use of time, let not advantage slip.

Chapter 8

Time's Edge: Leverage it for Success

In Health, as in Combat, Timing is of the Essence

Slim Samurai aims to make the case for the potential, demonstrate the practicality, and advocate for Judo-inspired strategies to tackle personal weight and energy regulation. In traditional Judo, as practiced in the combat arena, leverage over a formidable opponent is achieved through transfer-of-power tactics—redirecting an opponent's own force and momentum against them rather than opposing it directly. Analogously, I've argued that the most viable and practical approach to achieving *and* maintaining a healthy weight in today's obesogenic environment entails mastering two essential skills: (1) Developing a genuine, actionable understanding of the workings of our legacy (asymmetric) energy regulatory system; and (2) Applying that knowledge to devise personalized weight-management strategies that work *with* the body, not against it.

At its core, the "Judo way" espouses an *economy of means* mindset, which, I believe, is the ticket not only to successfully losing weight without undue hardship, but also to sustaining long-term weight loss. As the record clearly shows, living in an environment that consistently drives over-consumption of high-fat, high-calorie foods while fostering minimal physical activity, conventional "un-economy of means" weight-loss prescriptions often demand more willpower than people can sustain, inevitably leading to self-regulatory burnout—and relapse.

While we've already covered the nuts-and-bolts of *how* to formulate a Jugo-inspired personalized game-plan for losing weight, it is important to emphasize that *when* we act is just as crucial. Economy of means, in other words, is not just about how we accomplish things, but also about when we act. Indeed, the *how* and the *when* are inextricably linked, since what we can or cannot do at any moment is often constrained by decisions we've already made.

In combat Judo, timing is about seizing the opportune moment when the opponent is off-balance to make our move. I vividly remember from my Judo training how the coach would constantly drill into us that if our timing was too early or too late, the throw would feel like trying to move a mountain. But if the timing was perfect, he would often say, it would feel like moving a feather.

In this concluding chapter, I aim to persuade you that this principle is especially true when it comes to personal health regulation—including weight management. Specifically, delaying action to arrest or reverse gains in body weight—just like postponing interventions for many other health issues—can seriously aggravate and complicate the recovery task and increase the burden. To rephrase the coach: delay turns the weight-loss task from "moving a feather, to moving a mountain." Worse still, in matters of personal health regulation, delay often leads to adverse health consequences (as when delaying the removal of a precancerous colon polyp allows it to become cancerous). Human bioenergetics is no exception.

Surplus body fat, as noted in Chapter 1, is a metabolically active organ, producing hormones and chemical substances that can cause serious long-term damage. When excess body weight is allowed to accumulate and fester over an extended period, the cumulative stresses and collateral damage become increasingly difficult to reverse.[413] From a *Judo-esqe* perspective, it becomes harder because, as I explain below, entrenched (and possibly irreversible) physiological impairments make it more difficult for our body to work for us.

Unfortunately, many of us fail to fully appreciate the perils of delay and the critical importance of timely action when it comes to managing chronic health issues.[414] The reasons—and manifestations—are multiple and varied. In the case of body weight regulation, where weight gain typically occurs slowly over decades and adverse consequences are not immediate, I contend that a primary driver—a root cause—is human *maladaptation to slowly building threats*.[415]

This is an endemic, possibly ingrained, cognitive and behavioral predisposition that creates a significant vulnerability across a diverse range of human activities, not just body weight regulation. So, let's take a deep dive and try to better understand what it is and why it matters.

Specifically, I will seek to clarify three things:
- First, why it is relevant *here*
- Second, what *maladaptation to slowly building threats* means exactly, and
- Finally, the detrimental health consequences of delaying action

This nicely reconnects to the discussions and foundational concepts introduced in the opening chapters, allowing us to close the conceptual loop in the book's closing act.

It is Relevant *Here*... Because the Burden of Weight-Gain Builds Gradually Over Time

As discussed in Chapter 3, most people instinctively cruise on "automatic feeding control," instinctively regulating their feeding behavior in response to biological signals: eating when hungry, and stopping when full. While this "listen-to-your-body" instinct may have worked for our ancestors, it no longer serves us today. In our modern, food-rich, and activity-poor world, our legacy asymmetric system of energy regulation—evolved to favor over-consumption rather than under-consumption—is driving many of us to eat to our physiological limits, craving and prioritizing the abundant, energy-dense foods that are more affordable than ever. Meanwhile, a profusion of labor-saving devices reduces our physical exertion, prompting our bodies to store, rather than expend, the excess calories as body fat. The inevitable result is a persistent positive energy balance and an upward drift in body weight in a large proportion of the population.

What makes this dynamic particularly insidious, is that, for most individuals, weight gain tends to be slow and gradual enough to be easily dismissed. For example, the age-related upward drift in weight for adult men is, on average, only about half a pound per year.[416] And because there are often no *immediate* adverse consequences, the early stages of an expanding waistline usually go unnoticed or may be viewed as innocuous, inevitable, or even a sign of maturity.[417] As a result, the gradual increase in body weight may not be recognized until people find themselves trapped in an unhealthy, increasingly sedentary lifestyle, which can ultimately spiral into chronic obesity.[418]

In previous chapters, we saw how spiraling reinforcing processes can feed on themselves and amplify change—in a good way. For example, in Chapter 6, I discussed how these feedback processes can bolster our capacity to exercise: where exercising → enhanced physiologic capacity → enabling even more exercise. It is important to emphasize that such reinforcing feedback effects are neutral—"equal-opportunity" processes that are neither inherently good nor bad. In fact, the same self-reinforcing process can be virtuous—when it reinforces in a *desired* direction—or vicious

A familiar pocketbook example provides a clear illustration of this concept. Consider the dynamic between interest earned or owned and a cash balance in a bank. First, here's how compounding interest works in a virtuous self- reinforcing sort of way: A *positive* cash balance generates interest that is earned and reinvested → increasing the original principal → which in turn boosts the amount of interest that will be generated and reinvested the following year → and so on. Over time this makes us richer and richer (Figure 8.1, top half). Now, consider the different scenario of a bank balance that starts or turns negative—such as when taking out a bank loan say at a five-percent annual interest rate. The same compounding (snowballing) process now works in reverse: interest owed on the loan adds to the negative balance, increasing it and driving the account further into the red (Figure 8.1, bottom half).

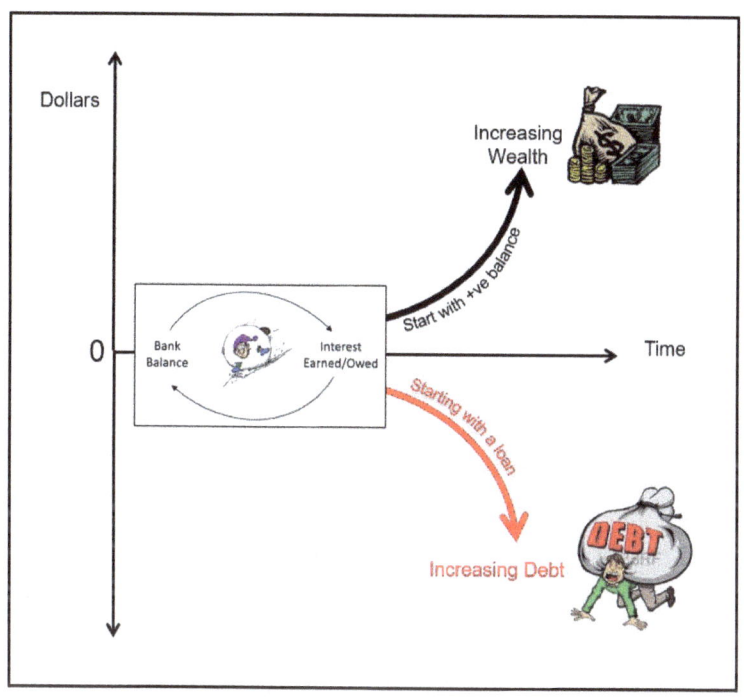

Figure 8.1
A reinforcing process can work virtuously or viciously

The "Dr. Jekyll and Mr. Hyde" characteristic of reinforcing loops applies to the health domain as well.

Here is how weight gain can transform the *virtuous* exercise loop from Chapter 6 into a *vicious* cycle: inactivity → diminished physiologic capacity to exercise and weight gain → fostering further decreases in activity → and ultimately, more weight gain. The primary reason why weight gain leads to less activity in this spiral is biological. Added pounds often trigger physiological complications—such as cardiovascular problems, respiratory difficulties, and osteoarthritis—that hamper a person's capacity to exercise.[419] But there's also a second, more sinister, non-biologic/cultural driver. It is sadly true that "among the most prevalent consequences of obesity, especially in children, is the discrimination they face from their peers."[420] Chubby children, for example, are less likely to be invited to participate in sports that leaner kids play. Exclusion can also be self-inflicted, as when an obese child chooses to voluntarily withdraw due to embarrassment. Either way, lack of participation robs overweight children (and adults) of the opportunity to practice and acquire skills, which accentuates their sporting ineptitude and leads to further exclusion—and more weight gain.

Bottom line: One of the ironies—and squandered opportunities—of the modern obesity epidemic is that while the effects of the mismatch between our (slightly) asymmetric system of energy regulation and our modern environment of abundance are small and *slow* to manifest—and should, in principle, be easier to tackle—they are proving to be quite the opposite. More vexing to mitigate.

But why? Why is it that, even as the pounds and the damage mount—albeit slowly—they often go unnoticed or are cavalierly dismissed?

Maladaptation to Creeping Threats

As noted in the book's opening, human beings are exquisitely adapted by evolutionary programming to recognize and respond to threats to survival that come in the form of sudden, salient events—such as a direct confrontation with a large predatory animal like a saber-toothed cat or a cave bear. However, slow and gradual change is less perceptible to our cognitive apparatus. (For example, a gradual decline in the population of prey species due to overhunting or increased human activity.) This phenomenon helps explain why we're more likely to notice signs of aging or senility in someone we don't see regularly—like distant relatives—than in a spouse or parent we see daily. In the case of weight gain, the slow, gradual updrift in weight—coupled with the lack of immediate adverse consequences—often keeps it off our RADAR.

Maladaptation to creeping threats has been so pervasive and enduring in human affairs that it has been enshrined in social and public policy circles as the "parable of the boiled frog" (discussed in the Prologue). The parable highlights how subtle, insidious gradual changes can go unnoticed and, even though they may be unhealthy or contrary to survival, can be tolerated over time, ultimately leading to harm for the unsuspecting or complacent.

Early in our evolution as a species, our alertness to jolting threats on the savannah provided a powerful advantage. Our predicament today is that the primary threats to our collective survival come not from sudden events but from slow, gradual processes.[421] The rise of religious militancy and the depletion of the ozone layer are slow, gradual threats. As is the growing obesity epidemic!

Warning: Delay in Action may be Hazardous to your Health

> *"Defer no time, delays have dangerous ends"*
> William Shakespeare

In the case of gradual weight gain, failing to recognize and respond in a timely manner means small gains will accumulate over a year, a decade, and a lifetime. The longer we wait to intervene, the more weight we gain, and the harder it becomes to reverse the damage. As I'll explain below, as surplus pounds accumulate over an extended period of time, the physiological stresses and consequences become increasingly difficult to undo.[422] It is not a matter of will—it's a matter of biology.

The biological and physiological underpinnings for why, were covered in Chapter 3. Delayed intervention to arrest or reverse weight gain obviously increases the risk of accumulating a larger weight burden. Since there are biologic limits to how much fat cells can expand, excessive weight gain inevitably triggers fat cell proliferation, thus increasing the body's stock of imperishable fat cells. The rise in the number of difficult-to-dispose fat cells, in turn, significantly complicates the task of reversing the weight gain. As discussed in Chapter 3, fat-cell theory suggests that an increase in the body's stock of fat cells ratches up the body's set-point—or physiologic target—for body weight. The increased number of fat cells, thus, results not only in an elevation of body weight but in the defense of that body weight.[423]

An instructive way to understand how this increases the body's resistance to weight-loss efforts is to think of physiological resistance in terms of *friction*. While the concept of friction originates in engineering, it applies broadly to all systems—mechanical, physiological, and even psychological. Fundamentally, friction is a force that resists or opposes movement or change, slowing us down or even halting us in our tracks when we try to move or alter something.

> [Friction is,] the thing that makes it harder for you to achieve your goal. Hence, reducing friction means removing an obstacle or coming up with a strategy that makes a task easier to do. And if you figure out how to make a goal easier, you're more likely to succeed.[424]

The proliferation of imperishable fat cells effectively builds up a form of biologic-type *friction* that opposes our efforts to shed surplus weight in two ways: (1) The increase in the stock of fat cells results in an elevation of the body's set point and the <u>defense</u> of that set point; and (2) these additional fat cells are next to impossible to dispose.

An increase in friction—whether it's the body's growing fat-preserving-defenses or, on a ski slope in the spring when rising water content makes the snow sticker and slower—slows us down and makes the task harder (Figure 8.2). As some of our energy is "spent" overcoming this friction rather than directly advancing our goal, the result is a decrease in efficiency. This is the antithesis of *Slim Samurai's* guiding principle of *Seiryoku-Zenyo*, or the efficient use of energy.

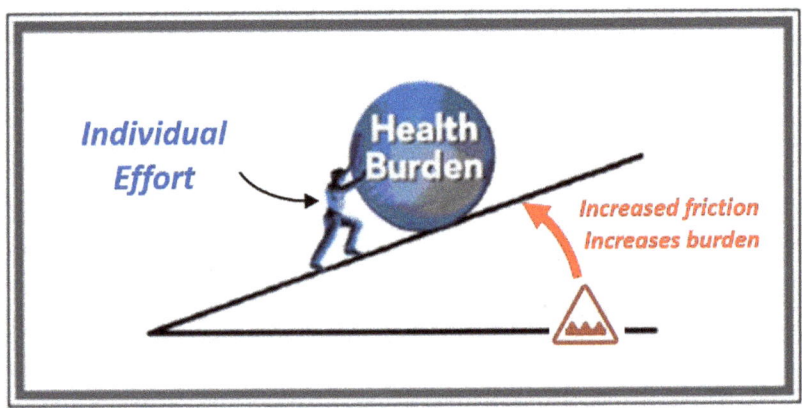

Figure 8.2
Increasing friction—like increasing the slope—increases burden

But the perils of delay go beyond just increasing the friction we face in trying to jostle our bodies back into shape. Delay also exacerbates the adverse health consequences that result from the cumulative stress of carrying excessive weight over an extended period. Wait too long, and you may very well reach a point where reversing the accumulated damage becomes impossible. If this sounds disheartening (or even heretical), it is understandable. America's popular and commercial cultures incessantly propagandize the seductive notion of our inexhaustible capacity for self-rejuvenation and self-repair. The promises are everywhere:

> (You) smoked? You can erase all those years of abusing your lungs if you just throw away the cigarettes. Eating a lot of junk food? Change your diet, lose even 5 or 10 pounds and rid yourself of those extra risks of heart disease and diabetes. Tan aficionado? (No worries) if you spent your youth in a state of bronzed bliss. Stay out of the sun—if you protect yourself now, skin cancer will never get you.[425]

In fact, science is pretty clear on all of this: There are real limits— and a steep price— when it comes to reversing the damage caused by a <u>lifetime</u> of unhealthy habits.[426]

Lifetime is underlined to underscore that timing is of the essence. Many adverse health consequences become increasingly harder to reverse as they become more entrenched.

Overweight is a prime example.

Gaining excessive weight, often as a direct result of delaying intervention, can induce a wide array of anatomic and physiological changes, some of which may lead to irreparable damage. For example, severe and persistent overweight is often associated with the buildup of plaque in the arteries and damage to blood vessels, contributing to coronary heart disease (CHD) and hypertension. Insulin resistance is another serious consequence of obesity, putting individuals at risk for Type 2 diabetes.[427]

However, these and other adverse health effects are easier to reverse when addressed early, before they become deeply entrenched. For example:

- **In type 2 diabetes,** ells that help regulate blood sugar stop functioning properly. While these cells were once thought to be permanently damaged, research now shows that some may recover—*especially with early intervention.*[428] Unfortunately, because insulin resistance often remains symptomless for years, intervention is frequently delayed, allowing elevated blood sugar to cause cumulative damage, sometimes with devastating consequences. **Déjà vu**—another case where acting sooner could have made all the difference.

- Similarly, advanced atherosclerotic lesions (plaque buildup in blood vessels) were once thought irreversible. However, recent studies suggest that *early-stage* lesions can, in fact, be reversed through cholesterol-lowering therapy.

The upshot of all this for personal health and weight regulation is clear: *don't delay*. Timely intervention not only makes reversing small weight gains easier, less costly, and more efficient, but it also helps avert the long-term health consequences caused by the cumulative stress of excess weight sustained over time.

Commander... and *Designer*

> *It is fruitless to manage an organization—or captain a ship—that is poorly designed.*
>
> Peter Senge,
> *The Fifth Discipline*, 1990

On several occasions in the book, I've likened the challenges of managing our bodies to commanding a ship on the high seas. Both are marvelously complex "machines," yet, both are highly vulnerable to turbulent environments—whether stormy or obesogenic. In either case, command and management are not a matter of making a single, one-time decision but rather a dynamic process involving a series of decisions made over time. Furthermore, the decisions are not independent of one another since what we can or cannot do now is often constrained by decisions we've already made.

The metaphor, while insightful, is not perfect however. Managing our bodies poses an added—and subtle—complication: we are not merely managing our them, we are also *redesigning* them as we go. Our bodies change continuously—autonomously (e.g., due to aging) and in response to the lifestyle choices we make each day. Managing our bodies, then, is akin to steering a ship through stormy seas while simultaneously redesigning and reconstructing it along the way. This dual role of commander and designer makes the challenge doubly complex—and often a frustrating.

It also makes the ability to regulate personal health both a perilous and fruitful endeavor—possibly flipping the script of Senge's cautionary quote above.

Perilous because delaying risks *self*-inflicting a wide array of physiological consequences that can lead to irreparable damage. Yet, **propitious** because acting expeditiously makes it easier for our body to work with us rather than against us. Early intervention prevents the escalation of the body's physiological friction or resistance, making the process of change smoother and more effective.

To vividly illustrate how advantageous it can be to leverage the capacity to *redesign* our bodies—both the target of and potential resistor to our efforts—let's don our metaphorical *Judogi* one last time! To a judoka, the fantastical capacity to reshape one's foe would be akin to facing a shape-shifting opponent that we can partially redesign (or shrink) mid-fight (Figure 8.3). Surely, that's a break that no judoka would sneer at. Dueling a diminished opponent would obviously be easier to handle and ultimately overcome. While we'd still need to apply leverage and technique to the fullest, using proper technique on a smaller opponent makes every judo throw or move more effective—essentially reducing friction and increasing the efficiency of each action we take.

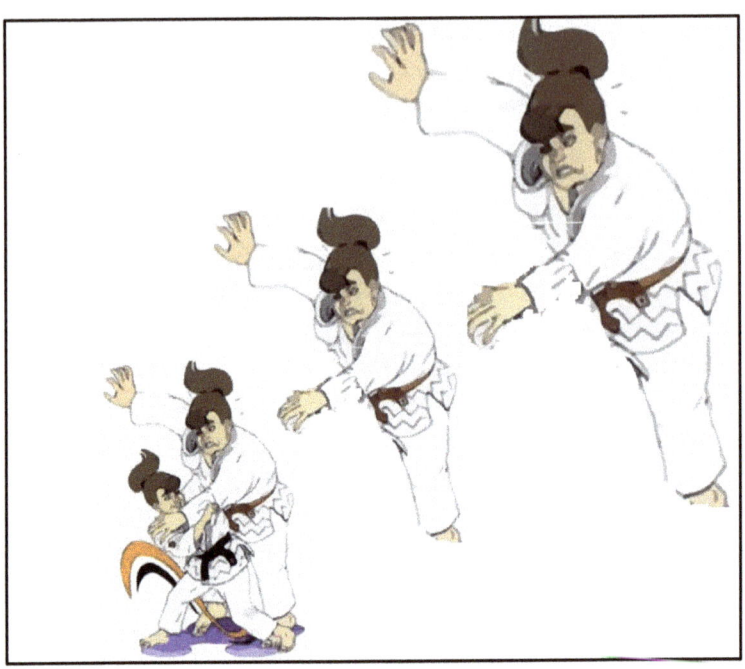

Figure 8.3
Diminishing Opponent

Conversely, delaying intervention to restrain or reverse incremental weight gain invariably ratches up the body's biological friction, effectively bolstering—rather than diminishing—the "physiologic foe." This can only exacerbate the hardship and increase the expense in time, effort, and financial cost required to shed the pounds and mitigate the damage.

As we wrap up, it seems fitting to leave you with Shakespeare's timeless insight, which I shared earlier: "Make use of time, let not advantage slip" (from *Richard III*). These words—circa 1592— still ring true, and we would be wise to heed his counsel and act accordingly.

INDEX

adipocytes, 53, 62
appetite regulation, 48, 51
   Long-Term Subsystem, 49
   Short-term Subsystem, 48
Asymmetry
   Asymmetry in Energy-Expenditure, 51
   Asymmetry in Energy-Input, 47
   Asymmetry in Energy-Storage, 53
body composition, 118, 119, 120
body mass index (BMI), 5, 8, 27
boiled frog, 6, 149
computer modeling, 121
computer simulation, 43
COVID-19, 6, 27
energy density, 61, 67, 71, 127
energy expenditure, 18, 46, 52, 118, 119, 125
energy intake, 40, 45, 47, 94
environment
   macro, 94
   micro, 95
environmental cues, 96
environments
   home, 96
evolution, 39, 44, 68
exercising, 122, 144
Exercising, 117
fast food, 115
fat cell theory, 56
fat mass, 118, 119, 120, 124

fat-free mass, 118, 120, 124
fatty foods, 65
Fatty foods, 40
feedback loop, 128, 144
friction, 150
ghrelin, 103, 126
glycogen, 133
goals, weight-loss, 135, 138, 139, 142
homeostatic processes, 14, 16, 54, 57
hunter-gatherer, 4, 41
illusion, 97, 99
Jigoro Kano, 32, 34, 35
judo, 32
Judo, 32, 36
K.I.S.S., 13
learning, genuine, 22, 23
leptin, 51, 59, 126
maintenance energy expenditure, 52, 120, 125
maximum-efficiency, 10, 18
mental models, 21, 22, 26
Mindfulness, 105
National Weight Control Registry, 29, 128
nonlinear, 138
obesity epidemic, 7, 114
Ozempic, 2, 13
passive overconsumption, 66, 115
positive-incentive theory, 57
reinforcing feedback, 144, 147

Reward of Food, 57
satiation margin, 71, 72
satiety signals, 50, 57, 59, 92, 98
Seiryoku-Zenyo, 31, 32, 129, 143, 150
self-efficacy, 15, 140, 142
self-regulation, 130, 140
SIGOS, 107
soft drinks, 67, 98
stock-and-flow, 131, 132
strength model of human self-regulation, 130

super-sizing, 102
tablescapes, 96, 99
thermic effect of food, 66
thermodynamics, 45, 62, 119
unique invulnerability, 8
unrealistic optimism, 7
weight-cycling, 27
wisdom of body, 25
yo-yo dieting, 142
Yo-Yo dieting, 19, 20, 138

Notes

[1] Walt, V. and Hirsch, L. (2023, September 4). The Disruptive Power of Weight Loss Drugs Is Being Felt Beyond Pharma. *New York Times*.

[2] Wilding, J. P. H, et al. (2021). Once-Weekly Semaglutide in Adults with Overweight or Obesity. *N Engl J Med*. 2021 Mar 18; 384 (11): 989-1002. (Wilding JPH, et al., Once-Weekly Semaglutide in Adults with Overweight or Obesity. *N Engl J Med.*, 384 (11), 989-1002.

[3] Gasoyan H, Pfoh ER, Schulte R, Le P, Rothberg MB. (2024). Early- and later-stage persistence with anti-obesity medications: a retrospective cohort study. *Obesity*. 2024;32(3):486-493.

[4] Pool, R. (2001). *Fat: Fighting the Obesity Epidemic.* Oxford: Oxford University Press.

[5] Koplan, J.P. and Dietz, W.H. (1999). Caloric Imbalance and public health policy. JAMA, 282(16), 1579-1581.

[6] Brownell, K.D. & Horgen, K.B. (2004). *Food Fight*. Chicago: Contemporary Books.

[7] Pool, R. (2001). *Fat: Fighting the Obesity* Epidemic. Oxford: Oxford University Press.

[8] Brownell, K.D. & Horgen, K.B. (2004). Food Fight. Chicago: Contemporary Books.

[9] Schlosser, E. (2002). Fast Food Nation: The Dark Side of the All-American Meal. New York: Perennial.

[10] Pool, R. (2001). *Fat: Fighting the Obesity Epidemic.* Oxford: Oxford University Press.

[11] Weigle, D.S. (1994). Appetite and the regulation of body composition. The FASEB Journal, 8, 302-310.

[12] Grundy, S.M. (1998). Multifactorial causation of obesity: implications for prevention. American Journal of Clinical Nutrition, 67(suppl), 563S-72S.

[13] Richmond, B. (1991). Systems thinking: four key questions. Hanover, NH: High Performance Systems, Inc.

[14] Senge, P.M. (1990). *The Fifth Discipline: The Art & Practice of the Learning Organization.* New York: Doubleday/Currency.

[15] Hogarth, R. (1987). *Judgement and Choice*. Chichester, NY: John Wiley & Sons.

[16] Senge, P.M. (1990). *The Fifth Discipline: The Art & Practice of the Learning Organization.* New York: Doubleday/Currency.

[17] Oliver, J.E. and Lee, T. (2005). Public Opinion and the Politics of Obesity in America. *Journal of Health Politics, Policy and Law*, 30(5), 923-954.

[18] Agrawal, N (2024, November 14,). Three-Quarters of U.S. Adults Are Now Overweight or Obese. *New York Times*.

[19] Huth, E.J. and Murray, T.J. (2000). *Medicine in Quotations: Views of Health and Disease through the Ages*. Philadelphia: American College of Physicians.

[20] Hammond, J.S, Keeney, R.L., and Raiffa, H. (1998). The Hidden Traps in Decision Making. *Harvard Business Review*, 76(5), 47-58.

[21] Hogarth, R.M. and Makridakis, S. (1981). Forecasting and Planning: An Evaluation. *Management Science*, 27(2), 115-138.
[22] Taylor, S.E. & Brown, J.D. (1988). Illusion and Well-Being: A Social Psychological Perspective on Mental Health. Psychological Bulletin, 103, 193-210.
[23] Whalen, C.K., Henker, B., O'Neil, R., Hollingshead, J., Holman, A., and Moore, B. (1994). Optimism in Children's Judgments of Health and Environmental Risks. Health Psychology, 13, 319-325.
[24] Taylor, S.E. & Brown, J.D. (1988). Illusion and Well-Being: A Social Psychological Perspective on Mental Health. Psychological Bulletin, 103, 193-210.
[25] Kuchler, F. and Variyam, J.N. (2003). Mistakes were made: misperception as a barrier to reducing weight. International J of Obesity, 27, 856-861.
[26] Etelson, D., Brand, D.A., Patrick, P.A., and Shirali, A. (2003). Childhood obesity: Do parents recognize this health risk? Obesity Research, 11(11), 1362-1368.
[27] Eckstein, K.C. et al. (2006). Parents' perceptions of their child's weight and health. Pediatrics, 117(3), 681-690.
[28] Klaas, B. (2024). *Fluke: Chance, Chaos, and Why Everything We Do Matters*. New York: Scribner.
[29] Peters, J.C., Wyatt, H.R., Donahoo, W.T., and Hill, J.O. (2002). From instinct to intellect: the challenge of maintaining healthy weight in the modern world. Obesity Reviews, 3, 69-74.
[30] Roy Bennett.
[31] Levitt, S.D. and Dubner, S.J. (2005). *Freakonomics: A Rogue economist explores the hidden side of everything*. New York: William Morrow.
[32] Polivy, J. and Herman, C.P. (2002). If at first you don't succeed: False hopes of self-change. American Psychologist, 57(9), 677-689.
[33] Wadden, T.A. & Stunkard, A.J. (Eds.). (2002). *Handbook of Obesity Treatment*. New York: The Guilford Press.
[34] Foster, G.D., Wadden, T.A., Vogt, R.A., and Brewer, G. (1997). What Is a Reasonable Weight Loss? Patients' Expectations and Evaluations of Obesity Treatment Outcomes. Journal of Consulting and Clinical Psychology. 65, 79-85.
[35] *Ibid.*
[36] *Ibid.*
[37] McArdle, W.D., Katch, F.I., and Katch, V.L. (1996). *Exercise Physiology: Energy, Nutrition, and Human Performance*. Baltimore, MD: Williams & Wilkins.
[38] Dansinger, M.L. et al. (2007). Meta-analysis: The effect of dietary counseling for weight loss. Ann Intern Med., 147, 41-50.
[39] Pi-Sunyer, F.X. (1999). Obesity. In M.E. Shils, J.A. Olson, M. Shike, and A.C. Ross (Eds.). *Modern Nutrition in Health and Disease*. Baltimore, MD: Williams & Wilkins.
[40] Shell, E.R. (2002). *The Hungry Gene: The inside story of the obesity industry*. New York: Grove Press.
[41] Hamid, T.K. (2009). *Thinking in Circles about Obesity: Applying Systems Thinking to Weight Management*. New York: Springer.

[42] Baumeister, R.F. & Heatherton, T.F. (1996). Self-Regulation Failure: An Overview. Psychological Inquiry, 7(1), 1-15.
[43] Blundell, J.E. & Tremblay, A. (1995). Appetite control and energy (fuel) balance. Nutrition Research Reviews, 8, 225-242.
[44] Shetty, P.S. (1990). Physiological mechanisms in the adaptive response of metabolic rates to energy restriction. *Nutrition Research Reviews* 3, 49-74.
[45] Parker-Pope, T. (2012, January 1). The Fat Trap. *New York Times*.
[46] Parker-Pope, T. (2011, December 28). The Fat Trap. *New York Times*.
[47] Mann, T., Tomiyama, A. J., Westling, E., Lew, A.-M., Samuels, B., & Chatman, J. (2007). Medicare's search for effective obesity treatments: Diets are not the answer. *American Psychologist, 62*(3), 220–233.
[48] Russo, E. (1990). *Decision Traps: The Ten Barriers to Decision-Making and How to Overcome Them*. New York: Fireside Publishing.
[49] Sterman, J.D. (2000). *Business Dynamics: Systems Thinking and Modeling for a Complex World*. Boston, Massachusetts: Irwin McGraw-Hill.
[50] Ann Chapman J. & Ferfolja, T. (2001). Fatal Flaws: The acquisition of imperfect mental models and their use in hazardous situations. *Journal of Intellectual Capital*, (2), 398-409.
[51] Sterman, J.D. (2000). *Business Dynamics: Systems Thinking and Modeling for a Complex World*. Boston, Massachusetts: Irwin McGraw-Hill.
[52] Ann Chapman J. & Ferfolja, T. (2001). Fatal Flaws: The acquisition of imperfect mental models and their use in hazardous situations. *Journal of Intellectual Capital*, (2), 398-409.
[53] Taylor, S.E. & Brown, J.D. (1988). Illusion and Well-Being: A Social Psychological Perspective on Mental Health. *Psychological Bulletin*, 103, 193-210.
[54] Peterson, C. & Stunkard, A.J. (1989). Personal Control and Health Promotion. Soc. Sci. Med., 28, 819-828.
[55] Sterman, J.D. (2000). *Business Dynamics: Systems Thinking and Modeling for a Complex World*. Boston, Massachusetts: Irwin McGraw-Hill.
[56] Sterman, J.D. (2000). *Business Dynamics: Systems Thinking and Modeling for a Complex World*. Boston, Massachusetts: Irwin McGraw-Hill.
[57] Whitney, E.N. and Rolfes, S.R. (1999). *Understanding Nutrition*. Belmont, CA: West/Wadsworth.
[58] Brownell, K.D. & Rodin, J. (1994). Medical, Metabolic, and Psychological Effects of Weight Cycling. *Arch Intern Med*, 154, 1325-1330.
[59] Hill, J.O. and Peters, J.C. (1998). Environmental Contributions to the Obesity Epidemic. *Science*, 280, 1371-1374.
[60] Wall Street Journal (2000, January 11). Being Overweight in Midlife Boosts Heart Risks. *Wall Street Journal*.
[61] Carlos Poston, W.S. and Foreyt, J.P. (2000). Successful management of the obese patient. *American Family Physician*, 61(12), 3615-3622.
[62] McKay, B. (2004, August 24). Obesity is linked to cancer risk. *Wall Street Journal*.

[63] Rabin, R.C (2020, October 14). Extra Pounds May Raise Risk of Severe Covid-19, *New York Times*.
[64] Wu, K.J. (2020, September 29). The Puzzle of Obesity and Covid-19. *New York Times*. page D4.
[65] *Ibid*
[66] Rabin, R.C (2020, October 14). Extra Pounds May Raise Risk of Severe Covid-19, *New York Times*.
[67] Brownell, K.D. & Horgen, K.B. (2004). *Food Fight*. Chicago: Contemporary Books.
[68] Brody, J. E. (2020, September 29). The Underused Weight Loss Option. *New York Times*, page. D7.
[69] Hill, J.H. and Wing, R. (2003). The National Weight Control Registry. *The Permanente Journal*, 7(3), 34-37.
[70] Senge, P.M. (1990). *The Fifth Discipline: The Art & Practice of the Learning Organization*. New York: Doubleday/Currency.
[71] Porter, R. ed. (1996). *The Cambridge Illustrated History of Medicine*. Cambridge, UK: Cambridge University Press.
[72] Lawrence, P.R. & Nohria, N. (2002). *Driven: How Human Nature Shapes our Choices*. San Francisco, CA: Jossey-Bass.
[73] Pool, R. (2001). *Fat: Fighting the Obesity Epidemic*. Oxford: Oxford University Press.
[74] Lawrence, P.R. & Nohria, N. (2002). *Driven: How Human Nature Shapes our Choices*. San Francisco, CA: Jossey-Bass.
[75] Lawrence, P.R. & Nohria, N. (2002). *Driven: How Human Nature Shapes our Choices*. San Francisco, CA: Jossey-Bass.
[76] *Ibid*.
[77] Eaton, S.B. (1992). Humans, Lipids and Evolution. *Lipids*, 27(10), 814-820.
[78] Pi-Sunyer, X. (2003). A clinical view of the obesity problem. *Science*, 299, 859-860.
[79] Peters, J.C., Wyatt, H.R., Donahoo, W.T., and Hill, J.O. (2002). From instinct to intellect: the challenge of maintaining healthy weight in the modern world. *Obesity Reviews*, 3, 69-74.
[80] Brownell, K.D. & Horgen, K.B. (2004). *Food Fight*. Chicago: Contemporary Books.
[81] Bray, G.A, Bouchard, C., and James, W.P.T. (Eds.). (1998). *Handbook of Obesity*. New York: Marcel Dekker, Inc.
[82] Wansink, B. and Huckabee, M. (2005). De-Marketing Obesity. *California Management Review*, 47(4), 6-18.
[83] Peters, J.C., Wyatt, H.R., Donahoo, W.T., and Hill, J.O. (2002). From instinct to intellect: the challenge of maintaining healthy weight in the modern world. *Obesity Reviews*, 3, 69-74.
[84] Brown, P.J. (1998). Culture, Evolution, and Obesity. In G.A. Bray, C. Bouchard, and W.P.T. James (Eds.). *Handbook of Obesity*. New York: Marcel Dekker, Inc.
[85] Pool, R. (2001). *Fat: Fighting the Obesity Epidemic*. Oxford: Oxford University Press.
[86] Bray, G.A, Bouchard, C., and James, W.P.T. (Eds.). (1998). *Handbook of Obesity*. New York: Marcel Dekker, Inc.

[87] Eaton, S.B., Eaton, S.B., Konner, M.J., and Shostak, M. (1996). An Evolutionary Perspective Enhances Understanding of Human Nutritional Requirements. *J. Nutr.* 126, 1732-40.
[88] Pool, R. (2001). Fat: Fighting the Obesity Epidemic. Oxford: Oxford University Press.
[89] The robber crab (birgus latro), shows amazing transitions between asymmetry and symmetry as adaptive responses to different stages of its life cycle. It begins its post-larval existence with a symmetrical abdomen. It then occupies a dextral gastropod shell (i.e. one with a left-banded spiral) and adapts to this change in habitat by developing an asymmetric abdomen. Once it has outgrown its adopted protective shell shelter and becomes free-living once more, it reverts back to its original symmetric design.
[90] Savage, S. (1998). Lecture at Stanford university.
[91] Abdel-Hamid, T.K.. (2012). EUREKA: Insights into Human Energy and Weight Regulation from Simple—Bathtub-like—Models. *Int. J. of System Dynamics Applications*, Volume 1, No. 3.
[92] Lawrence, P.R. & Nohria, N. (2002). *Driven: How Human Nature Shapes our Choices*. San Francisco, CA: Jossey-Bass.
[93] Lawrence, P.R. & Nohria, N. (2002). *Driven: How Human Nature Shapes our Choices*. San Francisco, CA: Jossey-Bass.
[94] Pool, R. (2001). Fat: Fighting the Obesity Epidemic. Oxford: Oxford University Press.
[95] Brownell, K.D. & Horgen, K.B. (2004). Food Fight. Chicago: Contemporary Books.
[96] Brownell, K.D. & Horgen, K.B. (2004). *Food Fight*. Chicago: Contemporary Books.
[97] Nielsen, S.J. and Popkin, B.M. (2004). Changes in beverage intake between 1977 and 2001. *Am J Prev Med*, 27(3), 205-210.
[98] O'Keefe, J.H. et al. (2010). Achieving Hunter-gatherer Fitness in the 21st Century: Back to the Future. *Am J Med*. 123(12):1082-6.
[99] *Ibid.*
[100] Dunn, D. (1997). Introduction to the study of women and work. In D. Dunn (ed.) *Workplace/Women's Place: An Anthology*. Los Angeles: Roxbury Publishing Company.
[101] Nestle, M. and Jacobson, M.F. (2000). Halting the obesity epidemic: A public health policy approach. *Public Health Reports*, 115, 12-24.
[102] French, S.A., Story, M., and Jeffery, R.W. (2001). Environmental influences on eating and physical activity. *Annu. Rev. Public Health*, 22, 309-35.
[103] Harris, L.M. (Ed.) (1995). *Health and the New Media: Technologies Transforming Personal and Public Health*. Mahwah, NJ: Lawrence Erlbaum Associates, publishers.
[104] Brownell, K.D. & Horgen, K.B. (2004). *Food Fight*. Chicago: Contemporary Books.
[105] Philipson, T.J. and Posner, R.A. (2003). The long-run growth in obesity as a function of technological change. *Perspectives in Biology and Medicine*, 46(3), S87-S107.
[106] Brownell, K.D. & Horgen, K.B. (2004). *Food Fight*. Chicago: Contemporary Books.
[107] Postrel, V. (2001, March 22). Americans' waistlines have become the victims of economic progress. *New York Times*, p. C2.
[108] Franklin, B.A. (2001). The downside of our technological revolution? An obesity-conducive environment. *The Am J of Cardiology*, 87, 1093-1095.

[109] Nestle, M. (2002). *Food Politics: How the food industry influences nutrition and health*. Berkeley, CA: University of California Press.
[110] National Institutes of Health (1998). *Clinical Guidelines on the Identification, Evaluation, and Treatment of Overweight and Obesity in Adults*. U.S. Department of Health and Human Services, NIH Publication No. 98-4083.
[111] Eaton, S.B., Eaton, S.B., Konner, M.J., and Shostak, M. (1996). An Evolutionary Perspective Enhances Understanding of Human Nutritional Requirements. J. Nutr. 126, 1732-40.
[112] Pool, R. (2001). *Fat: Fighting the Obesity Epidemic*. Oxford: Oxford University Press.
[113] Hargrove, J.L. (1998). Dynamic Modeling in the Health Sciences. New York: Springer.
[114] Koopmans, H.S. (1998). Experimental studies on the control of food intake. In G.A. Bray, C. Bouchard, and W.P.T. James (Eds.). Handbook of Obesity (pp. 273-311). New York: Marcel Dekker, Inc.
[115] Flier, J.S. and Maratos-Flier, E. (2007). What fuels fat. *Scientific American*, 297(3), 72-81.
[116] *Ibid.*
[117] Walsh, B.T. and Devlin, M.J. (1998). Eating Disorders: Progress and problems. *Science,* 280, 1387-1390.
[118] Shell, E.R. (2002). *The Hungry Gene: The inside story of the obesity industry*. New York: Grove Press.
[119] Whitney, E.N. and Rolfes, S.R. (1999). *Understanding Nutrition*. Belmont, CA: West/Wadsworth.
[120] Flier, J.S. and Maratos-Flier, E. (2007). What fuels fat. *Scientific American*, 297(3), 72-81.
[121] Bell, C.G., Walley, A.J., and Froguel, P. (2005). The genetics of human obesity. *Nature Reviews Genetics*, 6, 221-234.
[122] Rolls, B. (2007). *The Volumetrics Eating Plan*. New York: Harper Collins.
[123] Drenowski, A. and Specter, S.E. (2004). Poverty and obesity: the role of energy density and energy costs. *Am J Clin Nutr*, 79, 6-16.
[124] Rolls, B. (2007). *The Volumetrics Eating Plan*. New York: Harper Collins.
[125] Blundell, J.E. & King, N.A. (1996). Overconsumption as a cause of weight gain: behavioral-physiological interactions in the control of food intake (appetite). In Ciba Foundation Symposium ed. *The Origins and Consequences of Obesity* (pp. 138-154). Hoboken, NJ: John Wiley & Sons.
[126] Wansink, B. (2006). Mindless Eating: Why We Eat More Than We Think. New York: Bantam Books.
[127] Pollan, M. (2006). The Omnivore's Dilemma. New York: The Penguin Press.
[128] Peters, J.C., Wyatt, H.R., Donahoo, W.T., and Hill, J.O. (2002). From instinct to intellect: the challenge of maintaining healthy weight in the modern world. *Obesity Reviews*, 3, 69-74.
[129] Bjorntorp, P. (2001). Thrifty genes and human obesity. Are we chasing ghosts? *Lancet,* 358, 1006-1008.

[130] Russell, S.A. (2005). *Hinger: An Unnatural History*. New York: Basic Books.
[131] Jungermann. K. and Barth, C.A. (1996). Energy Metabolism and Nutrition. InR. Greger and U. Windhorst (Eds.). *Comprehensive Human Physiology*, (Vol.2, pp. 1425-1457), Berlin, Heidelberg: Springer-Verlag.
[132] Bjorntorp, P. (2001). Thrifty genes and human obesity. Are we chasing ghosts? *Lancet*, 358, 1006-1008.
[133] Bjorntorp, P. (2001). Thrifty genes and human obesity. Are we chasing ghosts? *Lancet*, 358, 1006-1008.
[134] Shell, E.R. (2002). *The Hungry Gene: The inside story of the obesity industry*. New York: Grove Press.
[135] Guyton, A.C. and Hall, J.E. (1996). *Textbook of Medical Physiology*. Philadelphia, PA: W.B. Saunders Company.
[136] Shell, E.R. (2002). *The Hungry Gene: The inside story of the obesity industry*. New York: Grove Press.
[137] Thorburn, A.W. and Proietto, J. (1998). Neuropeptides, the hypothalamus and obesity: insights into the central control of body weight. *Pathology*, 30, 229-236.
[138] Powell, K. (2007). The two Faces of fat. *Nature*, 447, 525-527.
[139] Woods, S.C., Schwartz, M.W., Baskin, D.G., and Seeley, R.J. (2000). Food Intake and the Regulation of Body Weight. *Annu. Rev. Psychol.* 51, 255-277.
[140] Mattes, R.D., Pierce, C.B., and Friedman, M.I. (1988). Daily caloric intake of normal-weight adults: response to changes in dietary energy density of a luncheon meal. *Am. J. Clin. Nutr.* 48, 214-9.
[141] Marx, J. (2003). Cellular warriors at the battle of the bulge. *Science*, 299, 846-849.
[142] Shell, E.R. (2002). *The Hungry Gene: The inside story of the obesity industry*. New York: Grove Press.
[143] *Ibid.*
[144] Whitney, E.N. and Rolfes, S.R. (1999). *Understanding Nutrition*. Belmont, CA: West/Wadsworth.
[145] Peters, J.C., Wyatt, H.R., Donahoo, W.T., and Hill, J.O. (2002). From instinct to intellect: the challenge of maintaining healthy weight in the modern world. *Obesity Reviews*, 3, 69-74.
[146] Polivy, J. and Herman, P. (1985). Dieting and Binging: A causal analysis. *American Psychologist*, 40(2), 193-201.
[147] Shetty, P.S. (1990). Physiological mechanisms in the adaptive response of metabolic rates to energy restriction. *Nutrition Research Reviews* 3, 49-74.
[148] Parker-Pope, T. (2012, January 1). The Fat Trap. New York Times.
[149] Pi-Sunyer, X. (2003). A clinical view of the obesity problem. *Science*, 299, 859-860.
[150] *Ibid.*
[151] McArdle, W.D., Katch, F.I., and Katch, V.L. (1996). *Exercise Physiology: Energy, Nutrition, and Human Performance*. Baltimore, MD: Williams & Wilkins.
[152] Dalton, S. ed. (1997). *Overweight and Weight Management: The Health Professional's Guide to Understanding and Practice*. Gaithersburg, Maryland: An Aspen Publication.

[153] Brownell, K.D. & Horgen, K.B. (2004). *Food Fight*. Chicago: Contemporary Books.
[154] Pool, R. (2001). *Fat: Fighting the Obesity Epidemic*. Oxford: Oxford University Press.
[155] McArdle, W.D., Katch, F.I., and Katch, V.L. (1996). *Exercise Physiology: Energy, Nutrition, and Human Performance*. Baltimore, MD: Williams & Wilkins.
[156] Whitney, E.N. and Rolfes, S.R. (1999). *Understanding Nutrition*. Belmont, CA: West/Wadsworth.
[157] Pi-Sunyer, F.X. (1999). Obesity. In M.E. Shils, J.A. Olson, M. Shike, and A.C. Ross (Eds.). *Modern Nutrition in Health and Disease*. Baltimore, MD: Williams & Wilkins.
[158] Whitney, E.N. and Rolfes, S.R. (1999). *Understanding Nutrition*. Belmont, CA: West/Wadsworth.
[159] *Ibid.*
[160] Pi-Sunyer, F.X. (1999). Obesity. In M.E. Shils, J.A. Olson, M. Shike, and A.C. Ross (Eds.). *Modern Nutrition in Health and Disease*. Baltimore, MD: Williams & Wilkins.
[161] Spalding, K.L. et al. (2008). Dynamics of fat cell turnover in humans. *Nature*, 453(7196), 783-7.
[162] McArdle, W.D., Katch, F.I., and Katch, V.L. (1996). *Exercise Physiology: Energy, Nutrition, and Human Performance*. Baltimore, MD: Williams & Wilkins.
[163] Fat cell size and number can be assessed from small tissue samples obtained (usually by means of a percutaneous needle aspiration) from multiple subcutaneous sites.
[164] Tate, D.F., Wing, R.R., and Winett, R.A. (2001). Using Internet technology to deliver a behavioral weight loss program. *JAMA*, 285(9), 1172-1177.
[165] Sjöström, L. (1980). Fat cells and body weight. In A.J. Stunkard (Ed.). *Obesity*. Philadelphia: W.B. Saunders Company
[166] Shils, M.E., Olson, J.A., Shike, M., and Ross, A.C. (Eds.). (1999). *Modern Nutrition in Health and Disease*. Baltimore, Maryland: Williams & Wilkins.
[167] Buckmaster, L. and Brownell, K.D. (1988). Behavior Modification: The state of the art. In R.T. Frankle and M. Yang (Eds.). *Obesity and Weight Control: The Health Professional's Guide to Understanding and Treatment*. Rockville, Maryland: Aspen Publishers, Inc.
[168] Vasselli, J.R. and Maggio, C.A. (1988). Mechanisms of appetite and body-weight regulation. In R.T. Frankle and M. Yang (Eds.). Obesity and Weight Control: The Health Professional's Guide to Understanding and Treatment. Rockville, Maryland: Aspen Publishers, Inc.
[169] There is now evidence that the induction of *ob* mRNA is a function of fat cell size, with larger fat cells expressing more *ob* mRNA than smaller cells. See: Jebb, S.A. et al. (1996). Changes in macronutrient balance during over- and underfeeding assessed by 12-d continuous whole-body calorimetry. *Am J Clin Nutr.*, 64, 259-66.).
Fat cell size may also be signaled through enzymatic mechanisms mounted on fat cell membranes. One such mechanism involves the enzyme lipoprotein lipase (LPL), which plays a key role in the process of lipid deposition in the adipose tissue. See: Whitney, E.N. and Rolfes, S.R. (1999). Understanding Nutrition. Belmont, CA: West/Wadsworth.
[170] Jéquier, E. and Tappy, L. (1999). Regulation of body weight in humans. *Physiological Reviews*, 79(2), 451-480.

[171] Whitney, E.N. and Rolfes, S.R. (1999). *Understanding Nutrition.* Belmont, CA: West/Wadsworth.
[172] Stipp, D. (2003, February 3). The quest for the antifat pill nature programmed us to overeat. Fen-Phen helped that, until it backfired. Safer drugs may be coming soon. *Fortune Magazine,* pp. 66-7.
[173] Buckmaster, L. and Brownell, K.D. (1988). Behavior Modification: The state of the art. In R.T. Frankle and M. Yang (Eds.). Obesity and Weight Control: The Health Professional's Guide to Understanding and Treatment. Rockville, Maryland: Aspen Publishers, Inc.
[174] Vasselli, J.R. and Maggio, C.A. (1988). Mechanisms of appetite and body-weight regulation. In R.T. Frankle and M. Yang (Eds.). *Obesity and Weight Control: The Health Professional's Guide to Understanding and Treatment.* Rockville, Maryland: Aspen Publishers, Inc.
[175] Mela, D.J. (2006). Eating for pleasure or just wanting to eat? Reconsidering sensory hedonic responses as a driver of obesity. Appetite, 47: 10-17.
[176] Cornier, M., Von Kaenel, S., Bessesen, D.H. and Tregellas, J.R. (2007). Effects of overfeeding on the neuronal response to visual food cues. Am J Clin Nutr, 86: 965–71.
[177] Bellisari, A. (2007). Evolutionary origins of obesity. Obesity Reviews, 9: 165-180.
[178] Cornier, M., Von Kaenel, S., Bessesen, D.H. and Tregellas, J.R. (2007). Effects of overfeeding on the neuronal response to visual food cues. Am J Clin Nutr, 86: 965–71.
[179] Heitman, B.L. and Garby, L. (2002). Composition (lean and fat tissue) of weight changes in adult Danes. Am J Clin Nutr, 75: 840-7.
[180] Pinel, J.P., Assanand, S. and Lehman, D.R. (2000). Hunger, Eating, and Ill Health. American Psychologist, 55(10), 1105 1116.
[181] *Ibid.*
[182] Pinel, J.P., Assanand, S. and Lehman, D.R. (2000). Hunger, Eating, and Ill Health. American Psychologist, 55(10), 1105 1116.
[183] Kessler, D.A. (2009). The end of overeating. New York: Rodale.
[184] Pinel, J.P., Assanand, S. and Lehman, D.R. (2000). Hunger, Eating, and Ill Health. American Psychologist, 55(10), 1105 1116.
[185] Pelchat, M.L. (2002). Of human bondage: Food craving, obsession, compulsion, and addiction. Physiology & Behavior, 76:347– 352.
[186] Erlanson-Albertsson, C. (2005). How Palatable Food Disrupts Appetite Regulation. Basic & Clinical Pharmacology & Toxicology, 97: 61–73.
[187] Saper, C.B., Chou, T.C. and Elmquist, J.K. (2002). The Need to Feed: Homeostatic and Hedonic Control of Eating. Neuron, 36:199–211.
[188] *Ibid.*
[189] Kessler, D.A. (2009). The end of overeating. New York: Rodale.
[190] Erlanson-Albertsson, C. (2005). How Palatable Food Disrupts Appetite Regulation. Basic & Clinical Pharmacology & Toxicology, 97: 61–73.
[191] Pinel, J.P., Assanand, S. and Lehman, D.R. (2000). Hunger, Eating, and Ill Health. American Psychologist, 55(10), 1105 1116.

[192] Flier, J.S. and Maratos-Flier, E. (2007). What fuels fat. *Scientific American*, 297(3), 72-81.
[193] McArdle, W.D., Katch, F.I., and Katch, V.L. (1996). *Exercise Physiology: Energy, Nutrition, and Human Performance*. Baltimore, MD: Williams & Wilkins.
[194] *Ibid.*
[195] Koplan, J.P. and Dietz, W.H. (1999). Caloric Imbalance and public health policy. *JAMA*, 282(16), 1579-1581.
[196] Drenowski, A. and Specter, S.E. (2004). Poverty and obesity: the role of energy density and energy costs. *Am J Clin Nutr*, 79, 6-16.
[197] Whitney, E.N. and Rolfes, S.R. (1999). *Understanding Nutrition*. Belmont, CA: West/Wadsworth.
[198] Rolls, B.J. (2009). The relationship between dietary energy density and energy intake. Physiology & Behavior; 97, *609–615.*
[199] Larkin, M. (2003). Can cities be designed to fight obesity? *The Lancet*, 362, 1046-1047.
[200] Hill, J.O. et al. (2003). Obesity and the environment: Where do we go from here? *Science*, 299, 853-855.
[201] Rolls, B.J. (2009). The relationship between dietary energy density and energy intake. Physiology & Behavior; 97, *609–615.*
[202] Blatt, A.D., Roe, L.S. and Rolls, B.J. (2011). Hidden Vegetables: An effective strategy to reduce energy intake and increase vegetable intake in adults. Am J Clin Nutrition, 93:756-63
[203] McCrory, M.A., Suen, V.M.M., and Roberts, S.B. (2002). Biobehavioral influences on energy intake and adult weight gain. The Journal of Nutrition, 132, S3830-S3836.
[204] Critser, G. (2003). Fat Land: How Americans became the fattest people in the world. Boston: Mariner Books.
[205] Popkin, B.M. (2007). The World is Fat. *Scientific American*, 297(3), 88-95.
[206] DiMeglio, D.P. and Mattes, R.D. (2000). Liquid versus solid carbohydrate: Effects on food intake and body weight. *International Journal of Obesity*, 24, 794-800.
[207] French, S.A., Story, M., and Jeffery, R.W. (2001). Environmental influences on eating and physical activity. *Annu. Rev. Public Health*, 22, 309-35.
[208] Schlosser, E. (2002). *Fast Food Nation: The Dark Side of the All-American Meal.* New York: Perennial.
[209] Critser, G. (2003). *Fat Land: How Americans became the fattest people in the world.* Boston: Mariner Books.
[210] *Ibid.*
[211] Taras, H. et al. (2004). Softe drinks in school. *Pediatrics*, 113(1), 152-154.
[212] Critser, G. (2003). *Fat Land: How Americans became the fattest people in the world.* Boston: Mariner Books
[213] Ludwig, D.S., Peterson, K.E., and Gortmaker, S.L. (2001). Relation between consumption of sugar-sweetened drinks and childhood obesity: a prospective, observational analysis. *The Lancet*, 357, 505-508.
[214] Brownell, K.D. & Horgen, K.B. (2004*). Food Fight*. Chicago: Contemporary Books.

[215] Wansink, B. (2006). *Mindless Eating: Why We Eat More Than We Think*. New York: Bantam Books.
[216] Koopmans, H.S. (1998). Experimental studies on the control of food intake. In G.A. Bray, C. Bouchard, and W.P.T. James (Eds.). *Handbook of Obesity* (pp. 273-311). New York: Marcel Dekker, Inc.
[217] Whitney, E.N. and Rolfes, S.R. (1999). *Understanding Nutrition*. Belmont, CA: West/Wadsworth.
[218] Anderson, G.H. (1993). Regulation of food intake. In M.E. Shils, J.A. Olson, and M. Shike (Eds.). *Modern Nutrition in Health and Disease* (8th edition). Philadelphia: Lea & Febiger.
[219] Baumeister, R.F., Heatherton, T.F., and Tice, D.M. (1994). *Losing Control: How and why people fail at self-regulation*. San Diego, CA: Academic Press.
[220] Blundell, J.E. & Tremblay, A. (1995). Appetite control and energy (fuel) balance. *Nutrition Research Reviews*, 8, 225-242.
[221] Baumeister, R.F., Heatherton, T.F., and Tice, D.M. (1994). *Losing Control: How and why people fail at self-regulation*. San Diego, CA: Academic Press.
[222] Capaldi, E.D. ed. (1996). *Why we Eat what we Eat: The Psychology of Eating*. Washington, D.C.: American Psychological Association.
[223] Blundell, J.E. (1995). The Psychbiological approach to appetite and weight control. In K.D. Brownell & C.G. Fairburn, C.G. (Eds.). *Eating Disorders and Obesity: A Comprehensive Handbook* (pp. 13-20). New York: The Guilford Press.
[224] Capaldi, E.D. ed. (1996). *Why we Eat what we Eat: The Psychology of Eating*. Washington, D.C.: American Psychological Association.
[225] Germov, J. and Williams, L. (1996). The epidemic of dieting women: The need for a sociological approach to food and nutrition. *Appetite*, 27, 97-108.
[226] Glanz, K., Rimer, B.K., Lewis, F.M. (Eds.). (2002). *Health Behavior and Health Education: Theory, Research, and Practice*. San Francisco, CA: Jossey-Bass.
[227] Forrester, J.W. (1979). System Dynamics: Future Opportunities. Paper D-3108-1, The System Dynamics Group, Sloan School of Management, Massachusetts Institute of Technology.
[228] Wansink, B. (2006). *Mindless Eating: Why We Eat More Than We Think*. New York: Bantam Books.
[229] Cornier, M., Von Kaenel, S., Bessesen, D.H. and Tregellas, J.R. (2007). Effects of overfeeding on the neuronal response to visual food cues. Am J Clin Nutr, 86: 965–71.
[230] Lowe, M.R. and Butryn, M.L. (2007). Hedonic hunger: A new dimension of appetite? Physiology & Behavior. 91, 432–439.
[231] Wansink, B. (2006). *Mindless Eating: Why We Eat More Than We Think*. New York: Bantam Books.
[232] Senge, P.M. (1990). *The Fifth Discipline: The Art & Practice of the Learning Organization*. New York: Doubleday/Currency.
[233] In 2017, red flags were raised/ criticism arose of the research methods and some of the findings in the published papers of Dr. Brian Wansink, who at the time was the head of Cornell University's Food and Brand Lab and is the former Executive Director of the

USDA's Center for Nutrition Policy and Promotion. The problems cited included data and figures being duplicated across papers, incorrect and inappropriate statistical analyses, and "p-hacking." As of 2020, Wansink has had 18 of his research papers retracted. After an announcement of his misconduct and resignation from Cornell, Wansink acknowledged in emails to Buzzfeed that there had been some problems with his publications but also wrote, "There was no fraud, no intentional misreporting, no plagiarism, or no misappropriation."

Much discussion and analysis has since followed... for and against. This author agrees with the sentiment that retraction of a journal article doesn't make its findings false. Wansink has published more than 500 articles. The retraction of eighteen papers—some of which have been replicated by others—is a blip receiving much more attention than his body of work deserves.

[234] Young, L. (2017). 8 Portion-Control Hacks That Really Work. This post was published on the now-closed HuffPost Contributor platform.

[235] Sobal, Jeffery and Brian Wansink (2007), Kitchenscapes, Tablescapes, Platescapes, and Foodscapes: Influences of Microscale Built Environments of Food Intake. *Environment and Behavior*, 39:1

[236] *Ibid.*

[237] Young, L. (2017). Moving Toward Mindful Portions in America. https://drlisayoung.com/wp-content/uploads/Portion-paper-NestleOct15.pdf

[238] Sobal, Jeffery and Brian Wansink (2007), Kitchenscapes, Tablescapes, Platescapes, and Foodscapes: Influences of Microscale Built Environments of Food Intake. *Environment and Behavior*, 39:1

[239] Wansink, B. (2006). *Mindless Eating: Why We Eat More Than We Think*. New York: Bantam Books

[240] *Ibid.*

[241] *Ibid.*

[242] Young, L. (2017). Moving Toward Mindful Portions in America. https://drlisayoung.com/wp-content/uploads/Portion-paper-NestleOct15.pdf chrome-extension://efaidnbmnnnibpcajpcglclefindmkaj/https://drlisayoung.com/wp-content/uploads/Portion-paper-NestleOct15.pdf

[243] Franklin, B.A. (2001). The downside of our technological revolution? An obesity-conducive environment. The Am J of Cardiology, 87, 1093-1095.

[244] Brownell, K.D. & Horgen, K.B. (2004). *Food Fight*. Chicago: Contemporary Books.

[245] Nielsen, S.J. and Popkin, B.M. (2004). Changes in beverage intake between 1977 and 2001. *Am J Prev Med*, 27(3), 205-210.

[246] Critser, G. (2003). *Fat Land: How Americans became the fattest people in the world*. Boston: Mariner Books.

[247] Brownell, K.D. & Horgen, K.B. (2004). *Food Fight*. Chicago: Contemporary Books.

[248] Brody, J.E. (2006, July 18). Wonder Where That Fat Cat Learned to Eat? *New York Times*.

[249] Spencer, M. (2004, November 7). Let them eat cake. *The Guardian Weekly*.

[250] Goode, E. (2003, July 22). The gorge-yourself environment. *New York Times*, p. F1

[251] Rolls, B.J., Engell, D., and Birch, L.L. (2000). Serving portion size influences 5-year-old but not 3-year-old children's food intakes. *J of the Am Dietetic Ass.*, 100(2), 232-234.
[252] French, S.A., Story, M., and Jeffery, R.W. (2001). Environmental influences on eating and physical activity. *Annu. Rev. Public Health*, 22, 309-35.
[253] Critser, G. (2003). *Fat Land: How Americans became the fattest people in the world.* Boston: Mariner Books.
[254] *Ibid.*
[255] Rolls, B.J., Engell, D., and Birch, L.L. (2000). Serving portion size influences 5-year-old but not 3-year-old children's food intakes. *J of the Am Dietetic Ass.*, 100(2), 232-234.
[256] Critser, G. (2003). *Fat Land: How Americans became the fattest people in the world.* Boston: Mariner Books.
[257] Rolls, B.J., Morris, E., and Roe, L.S. (2002). Portion size of food affects energy intake in normal-weight and overweight men and women. *Am J Clin Nutr*, 76, 1207-13.
[258] *Ibid.*
[259] *Ibid.*
[260] Young, L. (2017). Portion-Control Hacks That Really Work. This post was published on the now-closed HuffPost Contributor platform.
[261] Young, L. (2017). Moving Toward Mindful Portions in America. https://drlisayoung.com/wp-content/uploads/Portion-paper-NestleOct15.pdf
[262] Hazan, G. (2004, July 6). You are How you Eat. Giuliano Hazan. *New York Times.*
[263] Shell, E.R. (2002). *The Hungry Gene: The inside story of the obesity industry.* New York: Grove Press.
[264] Wansink, B. (2006). *Mindless Eating: Why We Eat More Than We Think.* New York: Bantam Books.
[265] Pollan, M. (2009). Food Rules: An Eater's Manual. London: Penguin Books.
[266] Hill, J.O. et al. (2003). Obesity and the environment: Where do we go from here? Science, 299, 853-855.
[267] Wansink, B. (2006). *Mindless Eating: Why We Eat More Than We Think.* New York: Bantam Books.
[268] Gordon, A. (2021). *The Way Out: A Revolutionary, Scientifically Proven Approach to Healing Chronic Pain.* New York: Avery.
[269] Taylor, V.A. et al. (2021). Awareness drives changes in reward value which predict eating behavior change: Probing reinforcement learning using experience sampling from mobile mindfulness training for maladaptive eating. *J Behav. Addict.* 10(3):482-497.
[270] Brewer JA, Ruf A, Beccia AL, Essien GI, Finn LM, van Lutterveld R and Mason AE (2018) Can Mindfulness Address Maladaptive Eating Behaviors? Why Traditional Diet Plans Fail and How New Mechanistic Insights May Lead to Novel Interventions. *Front. Psychol.* 9:1418.
[271] Parker-Pope, T. (2022, January, 4). Instead of Relying on Diets, Learn to Train Your Brain Instead. *New York Times.*
[272] Khare A and Inman J.J. 2009. Daily, Week-Part, and Holiday Patterns in Consumers' Caloric Intake. *J. of Public Policy & Marketing.* 28(2):234-252.

[273] Wansink B. 2004. Environmental Factors that Increase the Food Intake and Consumption Volume of Unknown Consumers. Annu. Rev. *Nutrition*, 24:455–79.
[274] Parker-Pope T. 2005. The Skinny on Holiday Weight Gain: It's Not as Bad as You Think, but it Sticks. Wall Street Journal, December 13; p. D1.
[275] Yanovski, J.A. et al. A prospective study of holiday weight gain. The New England J of Med. 2000; 342(12), 861-7.
[276] Cutler, D.M., Glaeser, E.L. and Shapiro, J.M. (2003). Why Have Americans Become More Obese? *Journal of Economic Perspectives*, 17(3), 93-118.
[277] Nestle, M. (2002). *Food Politics: How the food industry influences nutrition and health*. Berkeley, CA: University of California Press.
[278] Dunn, D. (1997). Introduction to the study of women and work. In D. Dunn (ed.) *Workplace/Women's Place: An Anthology*. Los Angeles: Roxbury Publishing Company.
[279] Cutler, D.M., Glaeser, E.L. and Shapiro, J.M. (2003). Why Have Americans Become More Obese? *Journal of Economic Perspectives*, 17(3), 93-118.
[280] Nestle, M. (2002). *Food Politics: How the food industry influences nutrition and health*. Berkeley, CA: University of California Press.
[281] Chou, S., Grossman, M. and Saffer, H. (2001). An economic analysis of adult obesity: Results from the behavioral risk factor surveillance system. *Third Int'l Health Economics Assoc. Conf.* York, England, Jul 23-25, 2001.
[282] Cutler, D.M., Glaeser, E.L. and Shapiro, J.M. (2003). Why Have Americans Become More Obese? *Journal of Economic Perspectives*, 17(3), 93-118.
[283] *Ibid.*
[284] Philipson, T.J. and Posner, R.A. (2003). The long-run growth in obesity as a function of technological change. *Perspectives in Biology and Medicine*, 46(3), S87-S107.
[285] Critser, G. (2003). *Fat Land: How Americans became the fattest people in the world*. Boston: Mariner Books.
[286] Bowman, S.A. et al. (2004). Effects of fast-food consumption on energy intake and diet quality among children in a national household survey. *Pediatrics*, 113(1), 112-118.
[287] French, S.A. et al. (2001). Fast food restaurant use among adolescents: associations with nutrient intake, food choices and behavioral and psychosocial variables. *International J of Obesity*, 25, 1823-1833.
[288] Bowman, S.A. et al. (2004). Effects of fast-food consumption on energy intake and diet quality among children in a national household survey. *Pediatrics*, 113(1), 112-118.
[289] Critser, G. (2003). *Fat Land: How Americans became the fattest people in the world*. Boston: Mariner Books.
[290] McCrory, M.A., Suen, V.M.M., and Roberts, S.B. (2002). Biobehavioral influences on energy intake and adult weight gain. *The Journal of Nutrition*, 132, S3830-S3836.
[291] French, S.A. et al. (2001). Fast food restaurant use among adolescents: associations with nutrient intake, food choices and behavioral and psychosocial variables. *International J of Obesity*, 25, 1823-1833.
[292] Cutler, D.M., Glaeser, E.L. and Shapiro, J.M. (2003). Why Have Americans Become More Obese? *Journal of Economic Perspectives*, 17(3), 93-118.
[293] *Ibid.*

[294] Kenney, J.J. (2004). To snack or not to snack, that is the question. www.foodandhealth.com.
[295] Zizza, C. et al. (2001). Sognificant increase in young adults' snacking between 1977-1978 and 1994-1996 represents a cause for concern! *Preventive Medicine*, 32, 303-310.
[296] Kenney, J.J. (2004). To snack or not to snack, that is the question. www.foodandhealth.com.
[297] McCrory, M.A., Suen, V.M.M., and Roberts, S.B. (2002). Biobehavioral influences on energy intake and adult weight gain. *The Journal of Nutrition*, 132, S3830-S3836.
[298] Franklin, B.A. (2001). The downside of our technological revolution? An obesity-conducive environment. *The Am J of Cardiology*, 87, 1093-1095.
[299] Brownell, K.D. & Horgen, K.B. (2004). *Food Fight*. Chicago: Contemporary Books.
[300] Pollan, M. (2003, October 26). The (Agri)Cultural Contradictions of Obesity. *New York Times Magazine*, p. 41.
[301] Martin, A. (2007, March 25). Will Diners Still Swallow This? *New York Times*.
[302] Rolls, B.J., Engell, D., and Birch, L.L. (2000). Serving portion size influences 5-year-old but not 3-year-old children's food intakes. *J of the Am Dietetic Ass.*, 100(2), 232-234.
[303] French, S.A., Story, M., and Jeffery, R.W. (2001). Environmental influences on eating and physical activity. Annu. Rev. *Public Health*, 22, 309-35.
[304] Drewnowski, A. (2003). Fat and Sugar: An economic analysis. *J. of Nutrition*, 133, 838S-840S.
[305] Shell, E.R. (2002). *The Hungry Gene: The inside story of the obesity industry*. New York: Grove Press.
[306] Story, M., Neumark-Sztainer, D., and French, S. (2002). Individual and environmental influences on adolescent eating behaviors. Supplement to the *J of the Am Dietetic* Ass, 102(3), S40-S51.
[307] Buckley, N. (2003, February 18). Unhealthy food is everywhere, 24 hours a day, and inexpensive. *Financial Times*, p. 13.
[308] Goode, E. (2003, July 22). The gorge-yourself environment. *New York Times*, p. F1
[309] Buckley, N. (2003, February 18). Unhealthy food is everywhere, 24 hours a day, and inexpensive. *Financial Times*, p. 13.
[310] Stipanuk, M.H. (Ed.). (2000). *Biochemical and Physiological aspects of Human Nutrition*. Philadelphia: W.B. Saunders Company.
[311] *Ibid.*
[312] Guyton, A.C. and Hall, J.E. (1996). *Textbook of Medical Physiology*. Philadelphia, PA: W.B. Saunders Company.
[313] Wadden, T.A. & Stunkard, A.J. (Eds.). (2002). *Handbook of Obesity Treatment*. New York: The Guilford Press.
[314] Bosy-Westphal. A. et al. (2009). Grade of adiposity affects the impact of fat mass on resting energy expenditure in women. *British Journal of Nutrition*, 101, 474–477.
[315] Westerterp, K.R., Donkers, J., Fredrix, E., and Boekhoudt, P. (1995). Energy Intake, physical activity and body weight: a simulation model. *British Journal of Nutrition*, 73, 337-347.

[316] Pi-Sunyer, F.X. (1999). Obesity. In M.E. Shils, J.A. Olson, M. Shike, and A.C. Ross (Eds.). *Modern Nutrition in Health and Disease*. Baltimore, MD: Williams & Wilkins.

[317] McArdle, W.D., Katch, F.I., and Katch, V.L. (1996). *Exercise Physiology: Energy, Nutrition, and Human Performance*. Baltimore, MD: Williams & Wilkins.

[318] Saris, W. H. M. Physical activity and body weight regulation. In: Regulation of Body Weight: Biological and Behavioral Mechanisms. C. Bouchard and G. A. Bray (Eds.). New York: John Wiley & Sons Ltd., 1996, pp. 135-148.

[319] Sterman, J. D. Business Dynamics: Systems Thinking and Modeling for a Complex World. Boston, Massachusetts: Irwin McGraw-Hill, 2000.

[320] Sterman, J.D. (2006). Learning from evidence in a complex world. *American Journal of Public Health*, 96(3), 505-514.

[321] Abdel-Hamid, T.K. (2003). Exercise and Diet in Obesity Treatment: An Integrative System Dynamics Perspective. *Medicine & Science in Sports & Exercise*, 35(3), 400-413.

[322] McArdle, W.D., Katch, F.I., and Katch, V.L. (1996). *Exercise Physiology: Energy, Nutrition, and Human Performance*. Baltimore, MD: Williams & Wilkins.

[323] Andrews, J. F. (1991). Exercise for slimming. *Proceedings of the Nutrition Society*. 50: 459-471.

[324] Melby, C.L., Commerford, S.R., and Hill, J.O. (1998). Exercise, Macronutrient Balance, and Weight Control. In D.R. Lamb and R. Murray (Eds.) *Perspectives in Exercise Science and Sports Medicine (Volume II): Exercise, Nutrition, and Weight Control*. Carme, IN: Cooper Publishing Group.

[325] Grundy, S. M., G. Blackburn, M. Higgins, R. Lauer, M. G. Perri, and D. Ryan. (1999). Physical activity in the prevention and treatment of obesity and its comorbidities: evidence report of independent panel to assess the role of physical activity in the treatment of obesity and its comorbidities. *Medicine & Science in Sports & Exercise*, 31: 1493-1500.

[326] Kirk, E.P., Jacobsen, D.J., Gibson, C., Hill, J.O., and Donnelly, J.E. (2003). Time course for changes in aerobic capacity and body composition in overweight men and women in response to long-term exercise: the Midwest Exercise Trial (MET). *International J. of Obesity*, 27, 912-919.

[327] The composition of weight loss is clearly a function of the type of exercise. Resistance training, for example, tends to preserve more of the fat-free mass component than does aerobic exercise.

[328] https://www.cdc.gov/healthyweight/physical_activity/index.html.

[329] Ballor, D.L. & Poehlman, E.T. (1994). Exercise-training enhances fat-free mass preservation during diet-induced weight loss: a meta-analytical finding. *International Journal of Obesity*, 18, 35-40.

[330] Gaesser GA, Angadi SS, Sawyer BJ. Exercise and diet, independent of weight loss, improve cardiometabolic risk profile in overweight and obese individuals. *Phys Sportsmed*. 2011 May; 39(2):87-97.

[331] https://www.cdc.gov/healthyweight/physical_activity/index.html.

[332] McArdle, W.D., Katch, F.I., and Katch, V.L. (1996). *Exercise Physiology: Energy, Nutrition, and Human Performance*. Baltimore, MD: Williams & Wilkins.

[333] Hill, J.O., Thompson, H., and Wyatt, H. (2005). Weight maintenance: What's missing? *Supplement to the J of the Am Dietetic Association*, 105(5), S63-S69.
[334] Stipanuk, M.H. (Ed.). (2000). *Biochemical and Physiological aspects of Human Nutrition*. Philadelphia: W.B. Saunders Company.
[335] Dullo, A.G., Jacquet, J., and Girardier, L. (1997). Poststarvation hyperphagia and body fat overshooting in humans: a role of feedback signals from lean and fat tissues. *J. Clin Nutr*, 65, 717-23.
[336] Heshka, S. Yang, M., Wang, J., Burt, P. and Pi-Sunyer, F.X. (1990). Weight loss and change in resting metabolic rate. *Am J Clin Nutr*, 52, 981-6.
[337] Saltzman, E. & Roberts, S.B. (1995). The Role of Energy Expenditure in Energy Regulation: Findings from a Decade of Research. *Nutrition Reviews* 53, 209-220.
[338] Sumithran P, Prendergast LA, Delbridge E, Purcell K, Shulkes A, Kriketos A, Proietto J. Long-term persistence of hormonal adaptations to weight loss. *N Engl J Med*. 2011 Oct 27: 365(17):1597-604.
[339] Parker-Pope, T. (2012, January 1). The Fat Trap. *New York Times*.
[340] Melby CL, Paris HL, Drew Sayer R, Bell C, Hill JO. Increasing energy flux to maintain diet-induced weight loss. *Nutrients*. 2019;11(10).
[341] *Ibid.*
[342] *Ibid.*
[343] Jebb, S.A. et al. (1996). Changes in macronutrient balance during over- and underfeeding assessed by 12-d continuous whole-body calorimetry. *Am J Clin Nutr.*, 64, 259-66.
[344] Wansink, B. (2006). *Mindless Eating: Why We Eat More Than We Think*. New York: Bantam Books.
[345] Kayman, S., Bruvold, W., and Stern, J.S. (1990). Maintenance and relapse after weight loss in women: behavioral aspects. *American Journal of Clinical Nutrition*, 52, 800-807.
[346] Brody, J.E. (2000, October 17). One-two punch for losing pounds: Exercise and careful diet. *New York Times*.
[347] Kessler, D.A. (2009). *The End of Overeating: Taking Control of the Insatiable American Appetite*. New York: Rodale.
[348] Brown, G. (1999). *The Energy of Life: The science of what makes our minds and bodies work*. New York: The Free Press.
[349] Polivy, J. and Herman, P. (1985). Dieting and Binging: A causal analysis. *American Psychologist*, 40(2), 193-201.
[350] Baumeister, R.F. & Heatherton, T.F. (1996). Self-Regulation Failure: An Overview. *Psychological Inquiry*, 7(1), 1-15.
[351] Blundell, J.E. & Tremblay, A. (1995). Appetite control and energy (fuel) balance. *Nutrition Research Reviews*, 8, 225-242.
[352] Muraven, M., & Baumeister, R. F. (2000). Self-regulation and depletion of limited resources: Does self-control resemble a muscle? *Psychological Bulletin*, 126, 247-259.
[353] Baumeister, R.F., Heatherton, T.F., and Tice, D.M. (1994). *Losing Control: How and why people fail at self-regulation*. San Diego, CA: Academic Press.

[354] Muraven, M., Tice, D. M., & Baumeister, R. F. (1998). Self-control as a limited resource: Regulatory depletion patterns. *Journal of Personality and Social Psychology*, 74, 774- 89.

[355] Muraven, M., & Baumeister, R. F. (2000). Self-regulation and depletion of limited resources: Does self-control resemble a muscle? *Psychological Bulletin*, 126, 247-259.

[356] Boekaerts, M., Pintrich, P.R., and Zeidner, M. (Eds.). (2000). *Handbook of Self-Regulation*. San Diego, CA: Academic Press.

[357] Boekaerts, M., Pintrich, P.R., and Zeidner, M. (Eds.). (2000). *Handbook of Self-Regulation*. San Diego, CA: Academic Press.

[358] Muraven, M., Tice, D. M., & Baumeister, R. F. (1998). Self-control as a limited resource: Regulatory depletion patterns. *Journal of Personality and Social Psychology*, 74, 774- 89.

[359] Tangney, J.P., Baumeister, R.F., and Boone, A.L. (2004). High self-control predicts good adjustment, less pathology, better grades, and interpersonal success. *J of Personality*, 72(2), 271-322.

[360] Baumeister, R.F., Heatherton, T.F., and Tice, D.M. (1994). *Losing Control: How and why people fail at self-regulation*. San Diego, CA: Academic Press.

[361] Muraven, M., Tice, D. M., & Baumeister, R. F. (1998). Self-control as a limited resource: Regulatory depletion patterns. *Journal of Personality and Social Psychology*, 74, 774- 89.

[362] *Ibid.*

[363] Muraven, M., & Baumeister, R. F. (2000). Self-regulation and depletion of limited resources: Does self-control resemble a muscle? *Psychological Bulletin*, 126, 247-259.

[364] Muraven, M., & Slessareva, E. (2003). Mechanisms of self-control failure: Motivation and limited resources. *Personality and Social Psychology Bulletin*, 29, 894-90.

[365] Muraven, M., Tice, D. M., & Baumeister, R. F. (1998). Self-control as a limited resource: Regulatory depletion patterns. *Journal of Personality and Social Psychology*, 74, 774- 89.

[366] Roizen, M.F. & Oz, M.C. (2006). *You on a Diet: The owner's manual for waist management*. New York: Free Press.

[367] Guyton, A.C. and Hall, J.E. (1996). *Textbook of Medical Physiology*. Philadelphia, PA: W.B. Saunders Company.

[368] McArdle, W.D., Katch, F.I., and Katch, V.L. (1996). *Exercise Physiology: Energy, Nutrition, and Human Performance*. Baltimore, MD: Williams & Wilkins.

[369] Roizen, M.F. & Oz, M.C. (2006). *You on a Diet: The owner's manual for waist management*. New York: Free Press.

[370] Freud, S. (1930). *Civilization and its discontents.* London: Hogarth.

[371] Tangney, J.P., Baumeister, R.F., and Boone, A.L. (2004). High self-control predicts good adjustment, less pathology, better grades, and interpersonal success. *J of Personality*, 72(2), 271-322.

[372] Muraven, M., Tice, D. M., & Baumeister, R. F. (1998). Self-control as a limited resource: Regulatory depletion patterns. *Journal of Personality and Social Psychology*, 74, 774- 89.

[373] *Ibid.*
[374] Muraven, M., & Baumeister, R. F. (2000). Self-regulation and depletion of limited resources: Does self-control resemble a muscle? *Psychological Bulletin*, 126, 247-259.
[375] Muraven, M., Tice, D. M., & Baumeister, R. F. (1998). Self-control as a limited resource: Regulatory depletion patterns. *Journal of Personality and Social Psychology*, 74, 774- 89.
[376] *Ibid.*
[377] Muraven, M. (2003). Blowing your diet: Models of self-control. *Contemporary Psychology*, 48(6), 742-44.
[378] Muraven, M., Tice, D. M., & Baumeister, R. F. (1998). Self-control as a limited resource: Regulatory depletion patterns. *Journal of Personality and Social Psychology*, 74, 774- 89.
[379] Tangney, J.P., Baumeister, R.F., and Boone, A.L. (2004). High self-control predicts good adjustment, less pathology, better grades, and interpersonal success. *J of Personality*, 72(2), 271-322.
[380] Muraven, M., & Baumeister, R. F. (2000). Self-regulation and depletion of limited resources: Does self-control resemble a muscle? *Psychological Bulletin*, 126, 247-259.
[381] Innate individual differences can now be measured. Tangney et al developed an instrument (based on 36 dimensions) to measure self-control strength. See: Tangney, J.P., Baumeister, R.F., and Boone, A.L. (2004). High self-control predicts good adjustment, less pathology, better grades, and interpersonal success. J of Personality, 72(2), 271-322.
[382] Muraven, M., Tice, D. M., & Baumeister, R. F. (1998). Self-control as a limited resource: Regulatory depletion patterns. *Journal of Personality and Social Psychology*, 74, 774- 89.
[383] *Ibid.*
[384] Muraven, M. (2003). Blowing your diet: Models of self-control. *Contemporary Psychology*, 48(6), 742-44.
[385] Muraven, M., Tice, D. M., & Baumeister, R. F. (1998). Self-control as a limited resource: Regulatory depletion patterns. *Journal of Personality and Social Psychology*, 74, 774- 89.
[386] Baumeister, R.F., Heatherton, T.F., and Tice, D.M. (1994). *Losing Control: How and why people fail at self-regulation.* San Diego, CA: Academic Press.
[387] Polivy, J. and Herman, C.P. (2002). If at first you don't succeed: False hopes of self-change. American Psychologist, 57(9).
[388] Kolata, G. (2007, May 8). Genes Take Charge, and Diets Fall by the Wayside. *New York Times.*
[389] Muraven, M., & Baumeister, R. F. (2000). Self-regulation and depletion of limited resources: Does self-control resemble a muscle? *Psychological Bulletin*, 126, 247-259.
[390] McArdle, W.D., Katch, F.I., and Katch, V.L. (1996). *Exercise Physiology: Energy, Nutrition, and Human Performance.* Baltimore, MD: Williams & Wilkins.
[391] *Ibid.*

[392] Armore, D.A. & Taylor, E.E. (1998). Situated Optimism: Specific outcome expectencies and self-regulation. In M.P. Zanna (Ed.), *Advances in experimental social psychology* (Vol. 30, pp. 309-379). New York: Academic Press.

[393] Polivy, J. and Herman, C.P. (2002). If at first you don't succeed: False hopes of self-change. *American Psychologist*, 57(9), 677-689.

[394] Baumeister, R.F., Heatherton, T.F., and Tice, D.M. (1994). *Losing Control: How and why people fail at self-regulation*. San Diego, CA: Academic Press.

[395] Polivy, J. and Herman, C.P. (2002). If at first you don't succeed: False hopes of self-change. *American Psychologist*, 57(9), 677-689.

[396] Whitney, E.N. and Rolfes, S.R. (1999). *Understanding Nutrition*. Belmont, CA: West/Wadsworth.

[397] Wadden, T.A. et al. (1992). Relationship of dieting history to resting metabolic rate, body composition, eating behavior, and subsequent weight loss. *Am J Clin Nutr*, 56, 203S-8S.

[398] O'Neil, J. (2003, October 7). For Youth, Downsize to Dieting. *New York Times*, p. D6.

[399] Field, A.E. et al. (2003). Relation between dieting and weight change among preadolescents and adolescents. *Pediatrics*, 112(4), 900-906.

[400] Polivy, J. and Herman, P. (1985). Dieting and Binging: A causal analysis. *American Psychologist*, 40(2), 193-201.

[401] Brownell, K.D. & Rodin, J. (1994). Medical, Metabolic, and Psychological Effects of Weight Cycling. *Arch Intern Med*, 154, 1325-1330.

[402] Kayman, S., Bruvold, W., and Stern, J.S. (1990). Maintenance and relapse after weight loss in women: behavioral aspects. *American Journal of Clinical Nutrition*, 52, 800-807.

[403] Whitney, E.N. and Rolfes, S.R. (1999). *Understanding Nutrition*. Belmont, CA: West/Wadsworth.

[404] Brownell, K.D. & Rodin, J. (1994). Medical, Metabolic, and Psychological Effects of Weight Cycling. *Arch Intern Med*, 154, 1325-1330.

[405] Kuhl, J, & Helle, P. (1986). Motivational and volitional determinants of depression: The degenerated-intention hypothesis. *J of Abnormal Psychology*, 95, 247-251.

[406] Brownell, K.D. & Rodin, J. (1994). Medical, Metabolic, and Psychological Effects of Weight Cycling. *Arch Intern Med*, 154, 1325-1330.

[407] Jairath, N. (1999). *Coronary Heart Disease & Risk Factor Management: A Nursing Perspective*. Philadelphia: W.B. Saunders Company.

[408] Glanz, K., Rimer, B.K., Lewis, F.M. (Eds.). (2002). *Health Behavior and Health Education: Theory, Research, and Practice*. San Francisco, CA: Jossey-Bass.

[409] Baumeister, R.F., Heatherton, T.F., and Tice, D.M. (1994). *Losing Control: How and why people fail at self-regulation*. San Diego, CA: Academic Press.

[410] Self-efficacy is not the same as self-esteem. Perceived self-efficacy is concerned with judgments of personal capability, whereas self-esteem is concerned with judgments of self-worth. Bandura (Bandura, A. (1997). Self-Efficacy: The Exercise of Control. New York: W.H. Freeman and Company) highlights the distinction between

the two concepts by pointing out that people can have high self-efficacy for a task from which they derive no self-pride (e.g., being able to brush one's teeth well) or have low self-efficacy for a task but have no loss of self-worth (e.g., not being able to ride a unicycle). However, he observes that people often try to develop self-efficacy in activities that give them a sense of self-worth, so that the two concepts are frequently intertwined (see, Strecher, V.J., DeVellis, B.M., Becker, M.H., and Rosenstock, I.M. (1986). The role of self-efficacy in achieving health behavior change. Health Education Quarterly, 13(1), 73-91.).

[411] Baumeiter, R.F. and Tierney, J. (2011). Willpower, New York: The Penguin Press.

[412] Dennis, K.E. and Goldberg, A.P. (1996). Weight control self-efficacy types and transitions affect weight-loss outcomes in obese women. *Addictive Behaviors*, 21(1), 103-116.

[413] Jeffery, R.W. (1998). Prevention of Obesity. In G.A. Bray, C. Bouchard, and W.P.T. James (Eds.). *Handbook of Obesity*. New York: Marcel Dekker, Inc.

[414] Plous, S. (1993). *The Psychology of Judgment and Decision Making*. New York: McGraw Hill.

[415] Senge, P.M. (1990). *The Fifth Discipline: The Art & Practice of the Learning Organization*. New York: Doubleday/Currency.

[416] Weigle, D.S. (1994). Appetite and the regulation of body composition. *The FASEB Journal*, 8, 302-310.

[417] Grundy, S.M. (1998). Multifactorial causation of obesity: implications for prevention. *American Journal of Clinical Nutrition*, 67(suppl), 563S-72S.

[418] Bjorntorp, P. (2001). Thrifty genes and human obesity. Are we chasing ghosts? *Lancet*, 358, 1006-1008.

[419] Mulvihill, M.L. (1995). *Human Diseases: A Systemic Approach*. Stamford, Connecticut: Appleton & Lange.

[420] Shils, M.E., Olson, J.A., Shike, M., and Ross, A.C. (Eds.). (1999). *Modern Nutrition in Health and Disease*. Baltimore, Maryland: Williams & Wilkins.

[421] Senge, P.M. (1990). *The Fifth Discipline: The Art & Practice of the Learning Organization*. New York: Doubleday/Currency.

[422] Jeffery, R.W. (1998). Prevention of Obesity. In G.A. Bray, C. Bouchard, and W.P.T. James (Eds.). *Handbook of Obesity*. New York: Marcel Dekker, Inc.

[423] Vasselli, J.R. and Maggio, C.A. (1988). Mechanisms of appetite and body-weight regulation. In R.T. Frankle and M. Yang (Eds.). *Obesity and Weight Control: The Health Professional's Guide to Understanding and Treatment*. Rockville, Maryland: Aspen Publishers, Inc.

[424] Parker-Pope, T. (2021) Erase Obstacles before creating new habits. *New York Times*. Jan. 19, 2021. P. D7.

[425] Kolata, G. (2005). The Body Heretic: It Scorns Our Efforts. *The New York Times*, April 17, 2005.

[426] *Ibid.*

[427] Hamid, T.K. (2009). *Thinking in Circles about Obesity: Applying Systems Thinking to Weight Management*. New York: Springer.

[428] Urbina, I. (2006, January 11). In the Treatment of Diabetes, Success Often Does Not Pay. *New York Times*.

About the Author

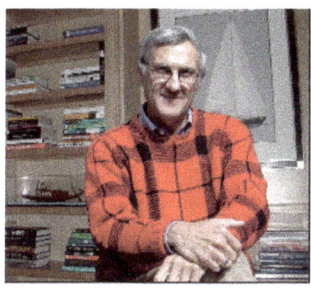

Dr. Tarek K.A. Hamid is a Stanford- and MIT-trained expert in system dynamics, with a deep interest in human metabolism and energy regulation. He holds a Master's from Stanford and a PhD from MIT and is a professor of System Sciences at the Naval Postgraduate School in Monterey, CA, where he received the Faculty Performance Award for excellence in research and teaching.

With a career spanning four decades, Dr. Hamid has applied systems thinking to a wide range of complex challenges—from NASA's project management practices to economic performance and, more recently, health and obesity. His interest in weight regulation took off in the mid-1990s when he recognized striking parallels between human metabolism and the kinds of feedback-driven systems he had spent years studying. This led him to further studies at Stanford, where he later became an affiliate of the university's Medical Informatics Department.

In 2009, he published *Thinking in Circles about Obesity* (Springer), an academic book exploring the obesity epidemic, which earned a "Highly Commended" distinction from the British Medical Association's Book Awards.

A few years later, he led the Systems Inspired Global Obesity Study (SIGOS), an international research effort involving scientists from seven countries. The study uncovered widespread misconceptions about weight gain, weight loss, and how people—both laypersons and healthcare professionals—misjudge obesity risks.

When he's not teaching or writing, Tarek enjoys sailing with his wife on their traditional Alden 45 sloop.

www.ingramcontent.com/pod-product-compliance
Lightning Source LLC
Chambersburg PA
CBHW041039050426
42337CB00059B/5062